CHRONIC FATIGUE SYNDROME

**A guide to the homeopathic treatment
of CFS/M.E.**

By Diane Solomon, B.S., DHM, Dip I.O.N.

Chronic Fatigue Syndrome: A guide to the homeopathic treatment of CFS/M.E.

by **Diane Solomon** B.S., DHM, Dip I.O.N. (London)

Eloquent Rascals Publishing
Hillsborough, NH

Website:
http://www.EloquentRascals.com

ISBN: 978-0-9907094-2-8

Disclaimer: The author is not a medical doctor. Nothing in this book is intended to diagnose, treat, cure or prevent *any disease.* The opinions expressed in this book reflect personal experiences and judgments based on practice, research and study.

This book is not a substitute for qualified medical advice, and does not provide guaranteed cures or fixes. You must not rely on the information in this book as an alternative to medical advice from your doctor or another healthcare provider. The author does not endorse or recommend any specific diet or food plan for therapeutic purposes.

The book contains general information about medical conditions and treatments. Nothing in the book is advice, and should not be treated as such. The author makes no representations or warranties in relation to the medical information in this book. Do not delay seeking medical advice or care, ignore medical advice, or stop medical treatment because of information in this book.

If you are pregnant, nursing, taking medication, or have a medical condition, be sure to consult your physician or qualified health practitioner before using any product.

DEDICATION

This book is dedicated, with love and empathy, to each and every soul struggling with Chronic Fatigue Syndrome. Although it has been called a life-destroyer, it does not have to be! It is not a "for life" jail sentence.

I know. I have been there, and returned to health to tell about it.

May you soon experience complete recovery! Here's to your total rejuvenation and restoration!

Table of Contents

PREFACE

With the wealth of available books discussing every possible factor relating to Chronic Fatigue Syndrome, you may wonder why I chose to write another one. I have studied this illness in the course of my practice as a nutritionist and homeopath and have information that may help. And, as a fully recovered CFS sufferer (a rare beast), I have a great deal of experience to share, and enormous understanding and compassion for anyone suffering this scourge.

I do not pretend that this is the be-all or end-all book on CFS, with regard to research, orthodox treatment, etc. There are high-quality books that lay out the history, symptomatology, CDC definition and treatment protocols, and possible alternative treatments. I simply put forward an overview of these areas. No need to re-create the wheel! However, few of these books touch on homeopathy in any in-depth way. In my opinion, having practiced for over 20 years, and worked with many CFS sufferers, homoeopathy is vital, even essential, to the treatment plan.

I wrote this book out of a passionate desire to help others afflicted by this syndrome, which stems, of course, from my own painful personal experience: seven devastating years of Chronic Fatigue Syndrome.

Here is a little of that story. I had completed my nutrition degree, in London, in 1986, from the Institute of Optimum Nutrition. I had practiced nutrition for some years, when I, of all people, came down with the dreaded Chronic Fatigue Syndrome, or Myalgic Encephalomyelitis, shortened to ME, as it is known in the UK. Imagine my shock, disbelief, and denial when I contracted what I thought was the flu, but never got better. It couldn't happen to *me*, I was a nutritionist! I ate organic food, drank very little alcohol, I exercised, I took tons of nutritional supplements. I was happy, having just fallen in love and was planning to move to Los Angeles to be with my fiancé.

Howeer, I had a history of Irritable Bowel Syndrome (IBS), and I needed to be very careful with wheat and other grains, all nuts, chocolate, and cheese. This was due to food intolerances or the tendency to the occasional migraine headache, inherited from my mother. So, I certainly wasn't able to lay claim to perfect health.

Stress had a great deal to do with it, too. I was selling my home in London, moving to California, planning my wedding, buying a home in Santa Monica, and my father was dying of pancreatic cancer. I flew from London to Los Angeles 22 times in 24 months, as well as making several trips to Massachusetts to see Dad. By the time he passed away, I was an exhausted wreck. Nutritional adrenal support helped a bit, then failed. Other energy nutrients and herbs didn't work. Rest didn't work. Exercise was impossible.

Sleep was elusive. I'd come down with the flu but didn't stop doing all the things that needed to be done. I worked and traveled right through it, out of sheer will power, and from a sense, however misguided, that it was absolute necessity that I do so. The Super Woman diagnosis definitely applied. I thought I could do anything.

Over the next seven years, I tried every possible modality. First, of course, were the orthodox physicians. Three of them. I heard "You're hyperventilating, breathe out of a brown paper bag and you'll be fine." This from an MD in England. "Try to get some more rest; here is a prescription for tranquilizers and sleeping pills." This advice from another general MD, this one in Los Angeles.

Then there was the MD at Cedar Sinai in Los Angeles who spent a great deal of the appointment time trying to persuade me to schedule a mammogram. (What did that have to do with the price of tomatoes that day?) I was there, desperate for help, with symptoms of systemic exhaustion, inflammation, swollen glands, sore throat, shaky feeling, weakness, foggy mental processes such as lack of concentration, and inability to sleep – all the symptoms of CFS. When I researched his clinic, I found that he part-owned the laboratory where he wanted to send me. Of course, this practitioner had nothing helpful to offer; he actually confessed he had no idea what was wrong with me. But he did present a large bill.

I also tried, oh, so many alternative practitioners, who, while more caring people, couldn't seem to help, either. I would find a bit of improvement from herbs, a chiropractic adjustment, acupuncture, or whatever, but it would not hold, and I'd sink right back down. I sought out naturopaths, acupuncturists, Chinese herbalists, chiropractors, a DO, massage therapy. I even tried hypnotherapy, in case I had somehow brought this all on myself and therefore my mind could undo it. I felt guilty contemplating that I had somehow done this to myself. But nothing I tried was of much use, certainly nothing lasting. I spent a fortune, was unable to work at the time, and was terrified. And very depressed about it.

The nutshell: years of bed-ridden misery. Sometimes I couldn't walk across the room unaided. I couldn't find the energy to answer the telephone. I couldn't sleep, so I never felt better in the morning. My first waking thought was "Oh my God, another day. How on earth do I get through it?" There was no reprieve from the never-ending headaches, body and muscle aches, and the inexplicable, all-consuming fatigue. Imagine you flew from L.A. to Bangkok (16 hours or so), with the flu, and a hangover, and then add the sensation that you've drunk five cups of coffee so you can't sleep. When you do sleep, it is a light, floating, semi-sleep full of horrible dreams, and you wake up over and over and over again. So the nights go on forever, but you feel no better in the morning. You just hurt all over like someone has hit you with a baseball bat about 40 times, and you honestly wish you were dead. That's Chronic Fatigue Syndrome.

It truly felt like a lifetime, these years of suffering, and thoughts of suicide haunted me. I know it was cowardice that prevented it, not any sense of hope. That was long gone.

Then I tried homeopathy – goodness knows why I did not find it sooner. A Los Angeles-based homeopath/Chinese herbalist recommended I take a nosode of Coxsackie B4 virus. (I know this may not mean much to you at this point – more later!) I took three doses over 24 hours and then promptly experienced a full-blown, terrifying relapse. Any tenuous balance or coping I was holding on to vanished with this remedy. I fell into bed – boy, did it ever make me sick! I was much worse; for about a week and a half I felt as if I had the full-blown flu. It scared me, I can tell you.

But then it was over. At about the ten-day mark, I just woke up. Everything felt different. There was no pain, no foggy feeling in the head, much less exhaustion, no swollen glands, no sore throat, no sore muscle points. I was still tired, weak, still had some mild IBS and gut problems, and the occasional inherited tendency to migraines that I had experienced for years before the CFS. But the majority of the symptoms were gone, and I was a consistent 80-85% better. No relapse. It took a while to clean up the gut, restore full adrenal function, and I was allergic to every food under the sun, it seemed, by this time.

There was more to do to be 100%. But, I felt like the black and white movie of my life had suddenly been re-mastered in gorgeous color. Like the curtains were raised. Like everything was in focus again. The fog and misery and aches and pains never returned. I was terrified that they might, for the next few years, but they never did.

Our belief, as homeopaths, is that my immune system was deeply challenged by the remedy of this virus (perhaps the virus of the original flu I had contracted seven years previously) and had kicked it out at last. The truth is, no one in the world of homeopathy knows exactly how this works, but that is my best guess.

I have since helped many people with CFS to recover some or most of their health with a remedy similar to Coxsackie. It might be another virus, such as Influenza or Cytomegalovirus, or even the Mononucleosis EBV virus. This is not to say that I think everyone with CFS will recover this dramatically with the use of a viral nosode, but it certainly can be a part of the picture needing to be addressed. Or, at least viral involvement must be eliminated as a cause.

That's a little of my story. I have been fully recovered now for over 20 years. I exercise, garden, hike, and ride my bicycle. I am back to normal, with a lingering mild problem with food allergies that I work on. Homeopathic desensitization techniques help, but have not completely eliminated the problem. And of course, I still have the occasional mild migraine. I have undergone constitutional treatment as well, and can honestly say I am healthier now than at any time of my life.

However, not a day passes that I don't feel truly blessed to have survived those dreadful years. When I get a cold or an occasional stress headache, I tell myself, "It's only a cold, it's not CFS," or "It's only a headache, it's not CFS." So it feels like nothing at all. Nothing could be that bad again, so this rebirth is just wonderful, just miraculous. A true gift!

I look at things differently now, I suppose not unlike those who approach death, yet escape. I am truly grateful that I didn't have the courage, all those years, to do the unthinkable. I am truly grateful that I am still here to enjoy my life, and that I might be able to help others who are lost and in pain.

If you enjoy this book, and find it useful, please consider posting a review on Amazon. Then I can reach even more people who may need this information. Thanks.

AMAZON REVIEW:

http://www.amazon.com/CHRONIC-FATIGUE-SYNDROME-homeopathic-treatment-ebook/dp/B0186JMJSC/

INTRODUCTION

Before discussing the treatment of Chronic Fatigue Syndrome (CFS), we must gain an understanding of this complex problem, within the limitations of what we know at the present time. Most people are now aware of CFS/ME, even though some may still think of it as the "Yuppie Flu." Most of us, unfortunately, know of someone with the illness. CFS is now estimated to affect approximately 2 - 4 million Americans and possibly 17 million people worldwide. Various epidemiological surveys find that between 1-3% of Americans are afflicted. A recent study showed that over 25 million Americans have severe fatigue, lasting at least one month at any time.[1] Approximately 85% of people with the disorder remain undiagnosed, so the true incidence of CFS is unknown. With all this variance, what is known is that this syndrome tends to hit people in their 40s and 50s, and occurs up to four times more often in women than men.

The definition of this illness, as set out by the Centers for Disease Control, in Atlanta, Georgia, has succeeded in setting guidelines for diagnosis. Although there is no accepted cure offered in the orthodox medical world, at least CFS is finally being accepted as a serious condition. Just this year, in February 2015, an Institute of Medicine report declared Chronic Fatigue Syndrome a "legitimate" illness, one that should be taken seriously by medical doctors. [2]

This will result, hopefully, in medical treatment aimed at a biological disease mechanism, not an emotional issue. Far too long CFS sufferers have had to contend with the "Yuppie Flu" brand, the depression misdiagnosis, or the "Oh, you're tired? I'm tired, too," comment from those who do not understand that having CFS is like living with a flu from which you never recover.

In a powerful turning point moment for the many sufferers of Chronic Fatigue Syndrome, a February 2015 Institute of Medicine news release stated, *"In its most severe form, this disease can consume the lives of those whom it afflicts. It is 'real.' It is not appropriate to dismiss these patients by saying, 'I am chronically fatigued, too.'"* [3]

The Institute of Medicine went on to recommend that Chronic Fatigue Syndrome be renamed "Systemic Exertion Intolerance Disease." Whether renamed or not, I am glad it will be reviewed and treated more seriously in the future.

There is research that points to possible markers for the disease, and which creates better understanding of what CFS does to the immune system and the nervous systems. However, this research has not yet led to much in the way of helpful orthodox treatment. In fact, it seems the drugs the medical world prescribes too often make a CFS sufferer feel even worse.

While I will attempt, in the appendices of this book, to lay out a general overview of the research and theories with regard to CFS/M.E., it is by no means complete. For the reader who wishes to read a summary and then move on to the homeopathic and complementary treatments of CFS, please check out Miriam E Tucker's succinct and thorough article for Medscape, which was published on January 8th of this year, 2015. It is entitled, *Chronic Fatigue Syndrome: Wrong Name, Real Illness.*

There are many current theories pertaining to possible causes of this syndrome. Perhaps part of the problem is that scientists and physicians are used to searching for a single cause, a smoking gun. They are looking to find a drug that will eradicate one invading organism, be it a virus, bacteria, parasite, fungus, etc. But, in the opinion of many experts and practitioners in the alternate and complementary health field, Chronic Fatigue Syndrome seems to be a plethora of problems piled high upon each other, and there is not one lone drug that holds the slam-dunk cure.

With this in mind, let's look at all the various indicating factors that may be involved in CFS. There is a high percentage of Chronic Fatigue Syndrome sufferers with what we call unresolved foci in the body, such as viral infection, parasites, dysbiosis (imbalance of the bacteria in the colon) and/or Candida inflammations of the bowel, and allergies to both foods and airborne substances. Many patients with CFS also have allergic or hypersensitive reactions to chemicals in the environment, heavy metal toxicity, thyroid toxicosis, and such problems as nutritional deficiencies. One or several of these problems may lead to an eventual diagnosis of Chronic Fatigue Syndrome, with the devastating fatigue, pain, and depression that this involves. It is important to use methods for diagnosing these problems, or foci, in order to unravel this syndrome.

The problems may be like an onion, in layers, which need to be peeled back. With the help of herbs, homeopathic remedies, and nutritional supplementation, much of the suffering involved in CFS can be dramatically alleviated, if not complete eradicated.

OVERVIEW

*"A CFIDS patient feels every day significantly the same
as an AIDS patient feels two months before death."*
Dr. Mark Loveless, infectious disease specialist at
Oregon Health Sciences University[4]

*"Chronic fatigue syndrome will be the dominant
chronic health disorder of the 21st century."*
Dr. Majid Ali, from *The Canary and Chronic Fatigue* [5]

Although Chronic Fatigue Syndrome has been the focus
of intense medical attention for only about 25 years, it seems
to be an old illness – an old illness that has had many names!
As early as the 1750s, a post-infection disorder was observed
by Sir Richard Manning, which he called "febricula." It later
came to be known as neurasthenia (exhaustion and
listlessness), atypical polio, "Royal Free disease," "endemic
neuromyasthenia" (USA), and Tapanui flu (New Zealand).
More recently it became known in the United Kingdom as
Myalgic Encephalomyelitis (this mouthful is fortunately
shortened to "M.E."), and chronic Epstein-Barr in the USA.

However, today it is primarily known as Myalgic
Encephalomyelitis (ME) in Great Britain, and Chronic
Fatigue Immune Dysfunction Syndrome (CFIDS), or just
Chronic Fatigue Syndrome (CFS) in the US. Arguing about
the proper name seems to me to be something of a waste of

resources, as CFS is now recognized by the World Health Organization as a "debilitating and distressing condition."

CFS: The CDC Definition

The CDC (Center for Disease Control in Atlanta, Georgia, in the USA) laid out its working definition of CFS (Holmes, et al) way back in 1994. (But, thanks to recent recommendations from The Institute of Medicine, this may be updated in the near future.) The consensus from the leading CFS researchers and clinicians is that Chronic Fatigue Syndrome is a subset of Chronic Fatigue, which of course is a broader category understood to mean prolonged fatigue. True CFS must be differentiated from prolonged fatigue.

Here are the official symptoms that must be evaluated to receive a diagnosis of CFS in America:

- Unremitting fatigue
- Sleep that is unrefreshing
- Muscle pain which is unexplained
- Poor concentration or loss of memory
- Sore throat
- Enlarged lymph nodes in armpits or neck
- A new type of headache, or headache that follows a new pattern or is more severe

- Joint pain that moves from joint to joint, with no redness or swelling
- Extreme exhaustion lasting at least 24 hours, following mental or physical exertion

The guidelines for evaluating CFS include a thorough medical history, physical exam, and lab tests before a diagnosis of CFS can be made. According to the CDC, clinically evaluated, unexplained chronic fatigue cases can only be classified as Chronic Fatigue Syndrome if:

Unexplained, persistent fatigue that is of new or definite onset (not lifelong), is not the result of ongoing exertion, is not substantially alleviated by rest, and results in substantial reduction in previous levels of occupational, education, social, or personal activities.

The concurrent occurrence of four or more of the following symptoms: substantial impairment in short-term memory or concentration; sore throat; tender lymph nodes; muscle pain; multi-joint pain without swelling or redness; headaches of a new type, pattern or severity; unrefreshing sleep; and post-exertional malaise lasting more than 24 hours.

These symptoms must have persisted or recurred during six or more consecutive months of illness and must not have predated the fatigue.

Furthermore, the CDC lists conditions that must be excluded or eliminated as a possibility before a diagnosis of CFS can be given.

Therefore, the practitioner must rule out infections, metabolic disorders, endocrine disorders, and cancer. He or she must exclude any other diagnosis that may explain the presence of chronic fatigue, such as untreated hypothyroidism (lowered thyroid function), sleep apnea and narcolepsy, and iatrogenic conditions such as side effects of medication. CFS must be differentiated from diagnosable illnesses that may relapse or may not have completely resolved during treatment, such as some types of malignances, hepatitis B or C virus infection.

Also major depressive disorders such as schizophrenia, dementia, bipolar affective disorder, etc, must be ruled out, as must alcohol or other substance abuse, or severe obesity.

The CDC does not condone batteries of tests other than those to exclude other medical explanations for the patient's fatigue. Only in the setting of protocol-based research is this suggested. These tests include serologic tests for Epstein Barr (over the history of ME/CFS this virus has been at times thought to be a prime indicating factor in CFS, and in 2014, evidence arose again for this theory), enteroviruses, retroviruses, human herpes virus 6, Candida Albicans, tests of immunologic function, including cell population and function studies, and imaging test such as MRI and radionuclide scans.

The CFS effect on lives

As you can see, CFS delivers a complex list of symptoms, primarily characterized by severe and lasting fatigue or tiredness. This fatigue is not relieved by rest or sleep, and is made dramatically worse by exertion or exercise. Patients suffering from this syndrome experience a drastically reduced level of activity. Many cannot work, or if they do, that's all they do. They go home so exhausted they can hardly function.

The sad list of symptoms is extensive. As well as the above characteristics, there is a variety of non-specific symptoms, including muscle aches or pains (fibromyalgia), malaise, weakness, headaches, sore throats, swollen and tender glands, intestinal complaints that resemble Irritable Bowel Syndrome, and recurrent low-grade fevers. Additionally, many CFS victims suffer from depression, insomnia and disturbed sleep, impaired memory and/or concentrations, visual disturbances, and vertigo.

The only way that CFS is currently diagnosed is by a history of illness based on the criteria of the CDC in Atlanta. This diagnosis is also dependent on the systematic exclusion of other possible causes of the symptoms. The patient must have experienced fatigue, plus a number of the other characteristic symptoms, for a minimum of six months.

CFS as a legitimate illness

*"I think the most important thing for physicians to
know is that while we don't have a diagnostic test
or a proven treatment, there is now abundant
evidence that in these [CFS] patients there is an
underlying biological process. Their symptoms are
linked to problems of their biology and not
imagined."* ~ Anthony L. Komaroff, MD, Harvard
Health Publications editor-in-chief.

This acceptance of Chronic Fatigue Syndrome as a
legitimate illness has finally given the CFS patient some
comfort. At least the illness has a name, and the sufferer no
longer feels so alone. After such a long period of being
diagnosed as having the derogatory "Yuppie Flu," or being
treated as having a psychosomatic illness related to stress, the
person in this position at least feels vindicated. He or she can
say, "See, I *told* you I was sick." However, this vindication
does not count for much when the patient realizes there is
little or nothing offered in the orthodox medical world that
will help.

And, strangely, there can be a distinct disadvantage to the
diagnosis and recognition of CFS as a true illness. After years
of denying its existence, allopathic medicine has finally
isolated the syndrome, given it a name, and relegated it to the
long, sad list of other chronic illnesses for which it has no
cure, only limited ability to alleviate symptoms.

A great disservice is done to this often-desperate patient by not searching further into his health problem. Rarely are stool samples taken, or digestive analysis carried out. No testing is done for heavy metals, or allergies, and of course, no suggestion is made that he see a homeopath, nutritionist, or any other holistic practitioner. So years can go by with little or no improvement in the health or standard of life of this patient, and he never knows, unless he delves into the world of alternative and complementary healthcare, that there is often help available.

Therefore, this disorder can persist indefinitely, since the medical orthodox establishment has, up until now, found no cause and few specific helpful tests to diagnose the condition. Furthermore, it has relatively little to offer in the way of treatment, except tranquilizers, anti-depressants, and/or anti-inflammatory drugs.

Fortunately, there are now signs that much of the medical and governmental world has recently begun to accept CFS as a genuine clinical condition, and there is new research, both clinical and epidemiological, being conducted regarding this devastating issue.

A Few Facts and Figures

- CFS is estimated to affect up to 2-4 million Americans[6] and up to 17 million people worldwide.

- Although there have certainly been "clusters" of CFS reported, such as the highly publicized outbreak in Lake Taho, Nevada between 1983 and 1986, there are no statistics that confirm that CFS is contagious. [7, 8] However, it sometimes occurs in the same family. This may be a genetic or familial link, which needs further research.

- It is estimated that up to 85% of Americans with CFS are undiagnosed.[9]

- Income level seems to play no part in who will come down with CFS.[10]

- CFS strikes more individuals in the USA than lupus, multiple sclerosis, and many types of cancer.[11]

- Women are more susceptible than men. [12]

- It is possible that only about 2% of CFS victims ever completely recover. [13] [14]

- Depression occurs for a percentage of those with CFS, but probably develops as a reaction to their poor quality of life and their frustration with an inability to recover. [15]

- CFS patients are significantly more likely to report a period of extreme stress or persistent nasal symptoms prior to the onset of the illness. [16] [17] [18]

- Chronic Fatigue Syndrome often seems to begin after an infection, such as influenza, or after a severe physical trauma or emotional shock. [19] [20]

- Some of the potential complications that accompany Chronic Fatigue Syndrome are depression, isolation, restriction of a normal lifestyle, and absence from work [21]

- The highest rate of recovery is in the first five years. Sudden onset patients have double the incidence of recovery than gradual onset patients. [22]

- A high proportion of CFS patients has neurally mediated hypotension, a defect in the way the body controls blood pressure [23] [24]

- In 80% of CFS sufferers, a crimson crescent can be seen over the uvula and tonsils, different from the

swelling and erythema of strep throat. [25] [26] [27]
(Although these crescents are also seen in many cases
of Mono, Lupus and Lyme Disease.)

- A large proportion of CFS sufferers has allergic
  reactions to many substances, and may even be so
  extreme as to be diagnosed as Multiple Chemical
  Sensitivity. These patients have severe reactions to
  perfumes, petroleum products, household chemicals,
  etc., as well as pollens, dust, molds etc. The majority
  of sufferers also react to some foods in an allergic
  manner, most often to wheat, grains and dairy
  products.

- Family studies of CFS patients point to an above
  average incidence of autoimmune diseases, allergies,
  and cancer [28] [29]

- Exercise exacerbates symptoms.[30] This distinguishing
  factor separates CFS from Fibromyalgia in diagnosis.
  Fibromyalgia patients tend to feel better from
  exercise, while those with Chronic Fatigue Syndrome
  are exacerbated by exercise. Patients report that the
  negative effects of exercise may take as much as
  several days to dissipate.[31]

- Several studies report immune system abnormalities
  which are suggestive of viral infection, such as a

decreased level of Natural Killer (NK)3 cell
function,[32] [33] [34] lowered tumor necrosis factor,[35]
atypical lymphocytosis, and both elevated and
reduced levels of Immunoglobulin G.[36] [37]

- At present, there is still no accepted specific
  biomarker for the diagnosis of CFS and its
  pathological fatigue.[38] There has been some work
  done investigating gene expression: a study in 2008
  found twelve genes, which were changed significantly
  in CFS patients.[39] But with regard to a single pathogen
  causing the syndrome, no evidence links any one virus
  or bacteria to CFS. For example, in 1997, a study
  published in Clinical Infectious Diseases compared
  CFS patients with healthy controls, looking for
  infectious agents. These were retroviruses,
  enteroviruses, arboviruses, Cytomegalovirus, Herpes
  Virus 6, Varicella Zoster, Epstein Barr, Hepatitis,
  Measles, Rubella, Parvovirus, Rickettsia, Candida,
  Chlamydia, and others. No evidence was found that
  the presence of any of these human pathogens
  increased the risk for developing CFS.[40]

- A possible marker may result from the latest research
  into spinal fluid of CFS patients. A clinical study,
  conducted by Dr. Mady Hornig of Columbia
  University, and published in the March 31, 2015 issue
  of *Molecular Psychiatry*, found that spinal fluid

samples from CFS sufferers showed reduced levels of
cytokines, and most specifically, eotaxin.
Interestingly, patients with multiple sclerosis shared
these raised levels of eotaxin cytokines. Dr. Hornig
explained that eotaxin is involved in immune
responses of the allergic type. These findings offer
hope that true biological markers may be established
for CFS sufferers, speeding treatment and acceptance.

- There is no evidence to support the theory that certain
  environmental or life-choice patterns put an individual
  at risk for developing CFS. In a 1996 study, there
  were no risk factors identified that effectively
  distinguish CFS from controls, having considered
  exposures to chemicals and sick animals, certain food
  consumption, allergies, travel, occupation, and
  recreational activity.[41] And the current CDC website
  confirms that besides the fact that CFS is more apt to
  hit adult women between 40 and 50, any other
  definitive risk factors are questionable. Further study
  is required to decide if it may be in some way a result
  of infections, immune disorders, stress, trauma, and/or
  toxins.[42]

ORTHODOX TREATMENT

The orthodox approach to the treatment of Chronic Fatigue Syndrome primarily consists of alleviating and suppressing symptoms.[43] These treatments have not substantially changed in the last twenty-five years, although they are only marginally effective. The patient's doctor may prescribe a variety of drugs, often off-label: antidepressants in low doses, such as Traxedone and Wellbutrin, Serotonin uptake inhibitors including Zoloft, Effezor and Prozac, central nervous system stimulants such as Adderall, and anti-virals such as Adamantane, to name but a few. All of these drugs have unpleasant side effects, and are of questionable value with CFS patients.

Anxiety medications such as benzodiazepines, which cause a dose-related depression of central nervous system activities, are sometimes prescribed for anxiety disorders. Adverse effects are plentiful. Another anti-anxiety drug is buspirone, which is similar to the benzodiazepines, and many adverse reactions have been reported to it as well. It does not help that these drugs are potentially addictive.

Anti-viral medication helps in some instances, such as for those patients who test positive for a certain type of herpes virus, known as chromosomally integrated HHV-6.[44] But because it seems to require a long time to see those

results, it is hard to conclude that this treatment is responsible
for the positive response. HHV-6 may be the cause of some
cases of CFS, but as yet we cannot say it is the single
causative factor. That still eludes researchers.

Non-sedating antihistamines are often prescribed for
relief of seasonal allergies (hay fever type symptoms), as CFS
patients have a higher tendency to develop allergies. Regular
antihistamines such as diphenhydramine and hydroxyzine are
also prescribed for allergic pruritis.

Immune suppressive drugs such as Azathioprine have
been tried by some physicians, but this is toxic to the immune
cells in the body. It is generally used to treat kidney transplant
patients to prevent organ rejection. This is experimental only,
and common sense tells us that depletion of immune cells
would lead to infection risks in an already compromised
individual. Severe nausea, vomiting, diarrhea, fever, skin
rashes, hair loss, are the side effects.

Researchers have even tried anti-cancer drugs,
cyclophosphamide and methotrexate, both of which are also
highly toxic to immune cells, and therefore are also
immunosuppressive. These drugs are also experimental, with
a long list of similar side effects to Azathioprine, above.

Among other miscellaneous therapies is Gamma
Globulin, its usage based on the unsubstantiated theory that
CFS is predominantly an underlying immune disorder.
Ampligen is a synthetic nucleic acid product tested in trial

with CFS patients, which stimulates the production of interferons, which are known to have anti-viral activity. Modest improvement has been reported in one study, and this treatment is considered experimental. Again, the participants in the trial reported adverse side effects.[45]

Another therapy tried is Kutapressin, a crude extract of pig's liver. This is also considered experimental, and there is as yet no clinical evidence of improvement using this extract. Other unusual experimental treatments for CFS are the use of pentoxifylline, a drug which lowers the viscosity of blood, presumably based on the idea that CFS sufferers have some cranial blood flow impairment. Adverse reactions include dizziness and gastrointestinal upset.

Another attempted drug treatment is the family of Beta blockers, such as atenolol, propranolol, betaxolol, etc., used in orthodox practice for the treatment of high blood pressure. As a large proportion of CFS patients seem to have an unusually low blood pressure, this would seem a less than successful choice. Side effects include slowed heart rate and headache.

Most recently, trials are ongoing using Rituximab a lymphoma cancer drug, being tried for symptom relief in CFS. Rituximab has shown success in this area, by suppression or elimination of B-cells in 67% of the patients in a 2011 trial, with another trial being carried out at the current time. (This is covered in greater detail in the appendix section entitled Rituximab Trials.)

All of these chemical drugs have great lists of adverse reactions, and interestingly, many alternate health practitioners and homeopaths have regularly reported that the CFS patients in their practices usually feel worse on any drugs or medications. Perhaps this is because they already suffer from a high level of toxicity, due to the disordered process of the body, and the chemicals add to this toxic burden.

THE HOLISTIC APPROACH:
Overview

Homeopaths, naturopaths, acupuncturists and other practitioners of alternate and complementary medicine do not put a lot of stock in the "single cause" theories for Chronic Fatigue Syndrome. With it encompassing such a complex group of symptoms, it just seems unlikely a "magic bullet" would be the answer (a cure-all that is intended to be effective in every case). Unfortunately, as well as the fact that most of the scientific world is searching for a single cause, it tends to believe that the human being, and indeed illness, follows a linear pattern. But "A" does not necessarily mean "B" in the course of ill health! Each patient is different. One person will cope adequately with a given stress or pathogen, while another will become chronically and desperately ill.

It is essential to treat each person individually, to search for the underlying causes of the illness, and eradicate them, whether they are viral, fungal, allergic, parasitic, etc. The person must be considered as a whole at all times. While I did work with people who, like I did, recovered dramatically with one remedy, generally this was not the case. It usually took tenacity and perseverance on my part, and on the part of the CFS sufferer.

In the alternative/complementary medical world, the emphasis is on getting the patient back in balance with nature.

This is the starting point. Benedict Lust, an American naturopathic doctor at the turn of the century said that one must, "eliminate the poisonous products in the system, and so raise the vitality of the patient."[46] It is difficult to imagine that the orthodox approach of adding drugs to a CFS patient's already toxic system would assist in this endeavor.

Whatever the approach or modality, the holistic practitioner tends to view Chronic Fatigue Syndrome as a complex matrix of symptoms with many different causes that vary greatly from individual to individual. Often there is a large stress component, coupled with something that may be called the "final straw." This consists of a viral, bacterial, or allergic attack that catapults the person into what has even been called "The Downhill Syndrome." Anything from a flu-like illness to severe stress to an exposure to a chemical such as new carpet, may be the "straw that broke the camel's back" in CFS. But, once again, it is important to remember that it is, after all, just the last straw. The secret is to search and "dig down" into the case to discover, then eradicate every toxin or focus.

Persons suffering from chronic illness rarely approach a homeopath, naturopath, or other complementary practitioner until much medical attention has been sought. (I often described my practice was "The House of Last Resort.") It is too often true that by the time the client finds a homeopath, all the other possibilities of cause of illness have usually been completed. If they have not, this needs to be addressed, as patients can be told they have Chronic Fatigue Syndrome when more diligent detective work and testing might have shown an amoeba infection, heavy metal toxicity, or root canal causing toxicity to the body. If this is the case, it is amazing how quickly a patient can "recover from CFS" with the correct treatment for the true cause of the condition.

Since definitions of Chronic Fatigue Syndrome list such a plethora of symptoms, it is possible for there to be other reasons for the complaints. Homeopaths, naturopaths, nutritionally oriented MDs, and other holistic health care professionals will employ nutritional supplements, herbal therapy, and homeopathic remedies to help their patients regain health. They will also suggest diet changes, saunas, colonic irrigation, acupuncture, therapeutic massage, psychological counseling, and many other means to detoxify, support, and rebuild the body and mind during its healing efforts.

In addition, the complementary practitioner may be more apt to offer a listening ear and even emotional support to the patient suffering from a debilitating illness. This alone can be a haven for the patient, who may have experienced a less than supportive atmosphere in his orthodox medical doctor's office.

HOMEOPATHY & CFS

"First and foremost, remove all obstacles to cure"
Dr. Samuel Hahnemann, 1755-1843, founder of Homeopathy

Homeopathic remedies play a powerful role in the treatment of Chronic Fatigue Syndrome. It is my opinion, supported by my years of clinical practice, that homeopathy is the most effective form of treatment for this devastating illness. Of course, it is also essential to use support, drainage, and terrain repair such as herbs, nutrients, exercise, and diet changes to help support the body through the healing process. Although in homeopathy we tend to rely on symptoms alone to choose remedies for our patients, it is also very helpful to have empirical, scientific data on our patients. In practice, we are greatly aided by blood tests, stool samples to diagnose parasites, heavy metal screening, etc. It is essential to use the largest arsenal of information we can!

I would venture to say that CFS is not brought about by single cause, i.e. virus, etc., but is a manifestation of the "onion layering" principle of ill health. This means there are often many contributing factors to an eventual diagnosis of CFS. Viruses, fungus, heavy metal toxicity, pesticide and chemical toxicity, dental focus such as root canal problems, nutritional deficiency, stress, and miasmatic influences can all play a part. Maybe there is no true Chronic Fatigue Syndrome, especially if one is searching for a single cause. Of course, one must remain open to the idea that some mitigating factor, which alters the immune system in some way, will yet be discovered. This remains to be seen, and research continues. But good homeopathic treatment, with nutritional support, will lead to dramatic improvement in most cases of Chronic Fatigue Syndrome.

Homeopathy:

Description and Background

Homeopathic philosophy is very different to that of orthodox medicine, as we know it. The orthodox medical world maintains an accent on finding a "single bullet' to attack any invader in the body. A good example is an antibiotic, which acts like a specific "hammer," targeting and killing specific bacteria. The body's own immune system does not take part in the fight, but is overridden by the antibiotic itself. In fact, the immune system is often suppressed during the duration of the course of antibiotic treatment.

When there is no single bullet available, the orthodox world tends to focus on the suppression of symptoms. Homeopathy, by contrast, sees the symptoms as the body's reaction against the illness as it attempts to overcome it, and seeks to stimulate, not suppress this reaction. It acts *with* the body, to raise its own defenses to battle the problem.

Therefore, the immune system takes part in the fight, and the body is stronger for it.

How does it do this? Homeopathy is a natural medicinal science that uses very small doses of plant, animal, or mineral substances to stimulate the body's innate healing ability. These are specially prepared, infinitesimal doses of substances that, in larger quantities, would cause the very symptoms they are trying to address. This basic principle has been known since the time of the ancient Greeks. Derived from the Greek word "Homoios' meaning "like," homeopathy is the practice of treating "like with like." Here's an example. When cutting onions for cooking, your eyes itch and run, your nose runs, and you sneeze. Onions made into a homeopathic remedy, known as Allium Cepa, can be very effective in reducing the symptoms of runny nose, itching eyes, and sneezing that accompany a cold or allergies. Another example is Poison Ivy (Rhus Tox). In homeopathic doses, Rhus Tox is a valuable remedy for certain skin rashes since in its undiluted state it causes them. Therefore "like cures like." This principle is known as the "law of similars," and has been used throughout history. Hippocrates himself wrote, "Through the like, disease is produced, and through the application of like it is cured."

Homeopathy was developed in the early 1800s by a German physician, Samuel Hahnemann. He was appalled by the medical practices of his day, and sought a method of healing which would be safe, effective, and gentle. During

this time cinchona (quinine) was established as the main
treatment for malaria. He discovered that taking a dose of
cinchona bark produced all the symptoms of malaria! But
when given to a patient suffering from malaria, it alleviated
the symptoms, and the patient recovered. Through his many
years of concentrated research he discovered many other
remedies, obtained from animal, vegetable, and mineral
sources that were just as effective in extreme dilutions. This
was apparent in the case of poison, which can produce
symptoms similar to those of certain illnesses. For example,
arsenic, in chemical dose, causes symptoms very similar to
food poisoning, or viral or bacterial gastroenteritis. In very
diluted doses, homeopathic doses, these substances can heal
on the "like cures like" principle, which is known as the Law
of Similars.

Samuel Hahnemann worked to establish the smallest
effective dose, realizing that his was the best way to avoid
side effects. In doing this he unexpectedly discovered that the
more a remedy is diluted, the more effective it becomes!
Since repeated dilutions cause the remedy to be more
powerful, or more potent, Hahnemann named this process
"potentization." With continued dilution, there comes a point
(beyond 24x or 12c) where the remedy no longer contains
even a single molecule of the original substance. Of course, it
seems impossible for remedies that contain no original
substance to have any effect. And, of course, this concept is
very foreign to today's scientific world. Physicians are taught
that drugs must be administered in sufficient doses to be

measurable in the blood. Hahnemann's findings contradict this.

No one can yet explain satisfactorily how homeopathic doses work. One theory is that succussion creates an electrochemical pattern somewhat akin to a holographic memory that is stored in the water and alcohol of the remedy and then spreads through the body's water. Another theory suggests that the dilution-succussion process creates an electro-magnetic field.

In any event, whatever the mechanism, there certainly is a difference between homeopathic remedies and water. Contrary to the claims of naysayers, there is a large body of laboratory evidence showing there IS a difference between homeopathic water and placebo water. In a 2007 review of 67 in-vitro studies, three-fourths of those have been replicated with positive results by independent investigators. The authors of the research review concluded, "Even experiments with a high methodological standard could demonstrate an effect of high potencies." Homeopaths hope this begins to lay to rest the whole "there's nothing in them" complaint which has plagued homeopathy to date.

Also, there have been careful double blind placebo studies to confirm the effectiveness of homeopathy, putting to rest the cry of "placebo effect" that the orthodox medical world has claimed.

In any event, homeopaths believe that these highly diluted doses of substances interact with the subtle energy system of the human body. It appears that water can be charged with subtle energies, and can store them. Interesting research has been conducted at McGill University in Montreal by Dr. Bernard Grad. Through a series of experiments using healers to "treat" water with the laying on of hands, he learned that the treated water was able to produce measurable changes in the growth and physiology of plants. Since the human body is made up of primarily water, it is possible that the homeopathy remedy interacts in some way with the water in the body, affecting change. It is theorized that homeopathic remedies are *frequency* matches to the frequency of the disturbance of the energy of the body.

Therefore, it seems most likely that Hahnemann was able to match the frequency of the substance with the frequency of the illness or symptoms. Taking the totality of symptoms, including emotional and mental states, as well as physical, allows for the closest possible match between the illness and the cure.

With modern physics constantly discovering smaller and smaller particles and their effects, and with the discovery that insects can detect and act on pheromones in the air to one part per million, the idea of an infinitesimal dose having an effect on the body no longer seems impossible.

Because they are so greatly diluted, homeopathic remedies are not harmful. They are not toxic, non-addictive, and therefore very safe. Homeopathic remedies, like all medicines, are regulated by the FDA. They will not interfere or react with other medications the patient may be taking.

Homeopathic remedies come in various forms, usually drops (water and alcohol), tablets, and pellets. They are best absorbed under the tongue, well away from food and drink. While taking remedies it is best to avoid caffeine, mint, menthol, camphor, and cortisone, as these substances will often antidote the remedies or lessen their effect in the body. The remedies must be stored away from magnets, microwave ovens, X-rays (care must be taken during air travel), heat over 150 degrees Fahrenheit, and strong smelling substances such as camphor and eucalyptus.

Having taken the homeopathic dose recommended by the practitioner, it is sometimes possible that the patient will experience an aggravation of symptoms before improvement begins. This is a confirmation that the correct remedy has been chosen, and is therefore not a negative reaction. However, it is also common for a level of relief to take place without this aggravation, and this of course is the ideal goal of the homeopath. Less is always better than more, when it comes to homeopathy, and when a reaction has taken place, it is usual to stop the remedy. For simple, acute conditions, it is fine to try homeopathic remedies on your own, but is best to work with a practitioner if you are dealing with more complex health issues and chronic complaints.

The deepest work in homeopathy is achieved through what is known as "miasmatic" treatment. A "miasm" is a predisposition to an inherited disease pattern, which can produce a tendency towards a variety of conditions. Hahnemann found several miasms that can be transmitted from one generation to another. One leads to disorders such as diabetes, insomnia, depression, alcoholism, osteoporosis, heart disease. Another leads to tendencies towards fibroids, cysts, tumors, asthma, allergies, and even manic depression. A third leads to eczema, psoriasis, one-sided migraines, anxiety. Miasms exist on very high vibrational levels, therefore miasmic treatment generally consists of higher and higher potencies, which go deeper and deeper into the systems to erase more and more of the miasmatic shadow, perhaps even the person's DNA.

When applied with wisdom, skill and experience, homeopathy instigates deep healing in the patient, while strengthening the immunity and vitality of the patient.

Classical Homeopathy & Homotoxicology

Classical, Kentian Homeopathy: There is an ongoing argument among the members of the homeopathic community with regard to the correct, most effective way to practice homeopathy. The Kentian school of classical homeopathy believes strongly in the use of one single remedy that most closely matches the patient's constitution, mental symptoms, physical general symptoms, modalities, etc., according to Hahnemanns's teachings. James Tyler Kent was a primary influence in homeopathic practice and theory in the later 1800s and early 1900s, and has remained so until today. At the time that Kent joined the ranks of homeopathy, it was a badly divided field. There were, essentially, the Hahnemannian purists, who rigidly adhered to the laws of Hahnemann and Hering. There were also those who more closely followed low-potency prescribing, and had a closer affinity for the world of orthodox medicine, claiming science as its principle and creed.

In his writings, Lectures on Homeopathic Philosophy, the Lectures on Homeopathic Materia Medica, and the Repertory to the Homeopathic Materia Medica, Kent's metaphysical outlook on homeopathy is clear. He insisted that homeopaths follow Hahnemann's theories, especially with respect to the vital force and doctrine of miasm. He placed the strongest emphasis on psychological and even spiritual prescribing. But unlike Samuel Hahnemann, his choice of remedies was always extremely high, using 30c only occasionally, but more often employing the M, CM, and even MM potencies, whereas Hahnemann rarely used higher than 30c. Finally, he rejected the concepts of the scientific and orthodox world of medicine as a means to prescribing.

Kent believed that homeopathy is founded in divine order and that disease results from sin against this order. Disease, to Kent, results from disorder at the inner levels of thinking and behavior. Therefore, he began to place the main emphasis of the selection of a remedy on the patient's mental symptoms. He took this trend very much further than did his mentor, Samuel Hahnemann. He wrote, in his Repertory, "Diseases correspond to man's affections, and the diseases that are upon the human race today are but the outward expression of man's interiors." and "The human race walking the face of the earth is little better than a moral leper." Moral standards, he felt, must be high in order to escape the ravages of disease, and respect for law and authority comes up again and again in the word "order." He had an invincible faith that he was right, even giving his followers the sense that to question Hahnemann was sacrilege.

Therefore, his teachings were in some ways the antithesis of science. Believing that homeopathy is metaphysical, even religious in nature, and a divine gift, he led homeopathic practice away from scientific principles of the day. And this he felt should be taken on faith. Although a respected, even idolized man, his writings, like those of Hahnemann, are often abusive to those holding opinions other than his own.

At the time of Kent, in England, Hughesian homeopathy was in the forefront, a pragmatic and non-metaphysical practice of homeopathy. It was situated at the "scientific" end of the homeopathic spectrum. Richard Hughes, and other leading British homeopaths, rejected the Hahnemann theory of the vital force, and placed little significance in the mental and emotional symptoms of the patient. Hughes, partly through his desire to unite homeopathy with orthodox medicine, espoused a form of homeopathy that employed low potencies- potencies that could be seen to have basis in science.

Hughesian homeopaths conceded that higher dilutions (up to 30c) did seem to have some effect, but were unhappy about being unable to explain this to the physicists, chemists, and orthodox physicians of the time. Therefore, the vast majority of British homeopaths used low material dilutions, 6c or below. However, Kent's philosophical ideas regarding homeopathy were extremely important and influential to the homeopathic community and Kentian philosophy remains the premier doctrine of the classical homeopath.

Not unlike the Hughesian followers of the turn of the last century, is a growing group of "homotoxicologists," those practitioners that employ low-potency remedies, often in combinations, known as complexes, to effect change on the body. The Italian, German, and French schools, particularly, use this method. Many of these practitioners respect and employ, when possible, a constitutional remedy along with lower potency remedies. They believe that there are pitfalls with the sole use of classical homeopathy. First of all, the practitioner must be very knowledgeable and skilled, and needs much previous experience to choose the correct remedy, in the correct potency, out of the many choices available. The process is based on matching the symptom pattern in the patient and the symptom pattern of the remedy, and knowing *which* symptoms in both are important for establishing the correct remedy.

Also, there is the great possibility of serious aggravation occurring with the initial dose of the constitutional, in a toxic system, which may have been weakened by the ravages of a serious illness such as Chronic Fatigue Syndrome. Perhaps LM potencies would solve this problem, but they are not at this time in common use by the homeopathic practitioner, and are not even readily available. Homotoxicologists like to "drain" the body, thereby lessening its toxic load, before attempting any deeper work such as the constitutional remedy. This will be gone into in more detail later; see the sections entitled Drainage and Support, Voll and Vega testing, Nosodes and Phases of Illness).

Both methods, classical and homotoxicolgy, are valid and useful. There are many practitioners today who employ the low-potency specific nosodes, drainage, and organotherapy as the initiating form of treatment, while using a high dose constitutional at the same time (or later) to work more deeply in the body. Unfortunately, there is still something of a rift between these two schools of thought, to the detriment of homeopathy around the world.

I do not doubt that the strictly classical approach works. I have just found that the quickest way to achieve results is to employ low-potency remedy combinations to drain and support the organ systems that are involved in the disease process. The patient simply feels better faster, without the chance of aggravation that one gets with the early use of the constitutional, even in a 30c potency. Perhaps LM potencies would solve this problem, but as yet I have not used them. In strict classical homeopathy, there is also the possibility that one will choose the remedy incorrectly. Without the use of Voll, Vega, or Kinesiology, this choice becomes even more dependent on the brilliance, experience and even intuition of the practitioner. When drainage and nosode work has been completed, the correct constitutional remedy can safely go deeper into the case, stimulating the patient's vital force, to address the reason he became ill in the first place. I find this the most judicious use of both systems of healing, in order to effect gentle, permanent, cure.

The true classical homeopathic purist argues that only one remedy must ever be employed at one time. Then it would stand to reason that the practitioner could only use, for example, the elemental minerals, not any combination of minerals. One must realize that many of our mineral remedies are combinations of two or even three minerals, such as Calcarea and Iodatum, forming Calcarea Iodatum, no longer a single substance. There are many other examples, including Kali Sulphuricum, Arsenicum Iodatum, Natrum Sulphuricum, and Aurum Muriaticum Natronatum (three substances combined).

In addition, to take this argument one step further, one must remember that a plant-based remedy, such as Pulsatilla, is made up of many constituents, as are all plants. Furthermore, various types of snake venom, when examined in laboratories, prove to be long chains of proteins that cannot easily be synthesized, as they are so complex.

Also, one must remember that we, as homeopathic prescribers, must remain open minded, which, after all, is a primary and fundamental requirement of all science. When we become rigid in our thinking, we become not unlike those in the orthodox medical community who will not even consider that homeopathy could possibly work. Hahnemann continued to experiment right up until the end of his life, and would have been "pushing the envelope" if he were with us today. As Dr. Richard Clements said recently at a BHI conference in New York City, "If Hahnemann were alive today, he'd have a website."

Furthermore, one must be wary of "belief." When an allopathic doctor states emphatically that he *believes* in orthodox medicine, the correct response from all true scientists would have to be "I do not operate from a place of belief. Belief has no place in science. In fact, belief is the absence of knowledge." That is to say, one must not be

blindly tied to one notion because one *believes* in it. This is
not the way of science, or indeed progress.

Drainage and Support

The first appropriate step in the treatment of the CFS
patient is thoroughly to take the case. This can take up to two
hours, and can tire the patient considerably. However, it is
essential to ascertain at least some previous history of the
person, to learn what his health was like before the onset of
the illness. One must know how the illness started, what
immediately preceded it, and, of course, the details of the
current symptoms. If the patient is extremely weak, it is
possible, perhaps preferable, to save the entire history (or the
homeopathic classical case-taking) until initial drainage work
has been undertaken. (See also the section entitled
Repertorization.)

Of course, to the classical homeopath, this is certainly
unconventional, as he or she swears by the prescription of one
lone single remedy. However, according to Dr. James
Compton Burnett, and my personal experience in clinical
practice, it is possible to severely aggravate the chronic
fatigue sufferer by too early administration of the
constitutional remedy, even in as low as a 30c. Therefore, it is
highly effective to employ, in Dr. Burnett's term,
"organotherapy" (low-potency drainage remedies and organ

support), before a homeopathic constitutional remedy is prescribed.

To quote Dr. Burnett, "In the acute processes, the value of a particular organ strikes one often very forcibly, there may be no need of any constitutional treatment; the one suffering part may be the whole case. And in many chronic cases certain organs claim and must have special attention... I do not regard organopathy as something outside Homeopathy, but as being embraced by, and included in it, or co-extensive with it. I would say Organopathy is Homeopathy in the first degree."

Homeopathic organ support and drainage with Mother Tinctures, herbs, and low-potency homeopathic remedies has many benefits to the patient. It increases the activity of excretory organs and the biological flow in the connective tissue in order to create cleansing. The organs are able to detoxify, with the help of drainage remedies to aid them in the elimination process. Through this stimulation or regulation of the organ, congestion is eliminated through re-absorption.

For example, the kidneys can be drained, or detoxified by the help of Berberis Vulgaris (MT, 1x or 3x), so that the kidneys can more readily excrete toxins, pollutants, and debris of metabolic processes through the urine. Drainage also can help to clarify the symptom picture. As the toxification symptoms are reduced, a clearer picture of the underlying problem begins to emerge. In addition, using drainage remedies helps the patient to feel better quickly. It can be very advantageous to use drainage *before* constitutional treatment in order that the organs are stronger, healthier, and less toxic. There is less strain on the system if it is cleared of some of the toxicity before nosode or constitutional work is begun. This means there can be far less chance of aggravation when the constitutional remedy is prescribed. Drainage remedies are safe, gentle, and can even promote spontaneous healing. When the toxins are removed from the body, often "the doctor within" (the body's innate ability to heal and balance itself) can begin the healing.

The patient must remember there will often be a "healing crisis" in this drainage period, and know how to proceed if this occurs. Acute inflammation is appropriate for the body, in that it is the expression of the body detoxifying itself. So to this end it should not be suppressed, as per the orthodox medical establishment, which fights illness with *anti*biotic, *anti*pyretic, *anti*-diarrheal, and *anti*-inflammatory drugs. However, it is not necessary that the patient experiences severe symptoms, as this can indeed be very tiring to a weakened system. Therefore, it is a good idea for him to take a couple of days off the drainage remedies if the reaction is strong, to allow some natural clearing and settling of the system. It is very helpful to take several grams of Vitamin C per day (e.g., Calcium Ascorbate, 8 x 500 mg capsules), and to drink plenty of pure water to aid the detoxification process.

EAV / Voll Testing

In order to decide upon the drainage and organ therapy remedies, it can be helpful to utilize Electrodermal Screening. This is the umbrella term that includes Electroacupuncture according to Voll, Vegatest, and computerized screening with Listen System, etc. As a practitioner of EAV, (Electroacupuncture According to Voll), I found it very useful. One can very quickly and easily learn a great deal about the state of the patient: which organ systems are the most involved, the state of inflammation in the lymphatic system, and the strength of the patient's vital force.

Electrodermal Screening tests the subtle energies that flow through the meridian channels of the body. These meridian channels provide us with acupuncture points that can reveal information about the body's internal organs.

Electroacupuncture, sometimes called EAP, or EAV (Electroacupuncture according to Voll) is based on the traditional Chinese acupuncture meridian system, in conjunction with modern electronic circuits. It is able to measure the electrical parameters of any acupuncture point on the body.

Electroacupuncture was developed by a German physician, Dr. Rheinhold Voll, in 1953. A high precision ohmmeter is used to measure the resistance of human skin. This, along with measurements at specific points of meridian channels of the body, can exactly determine the energetic potential of each organ. The patient holds a brass electrode (negative) while the practitioner makes contact to the specific points, most often located on the fingers and toes, with his hand-held positively charged electrode. The normal healthy reading for these points is 50. An inflammation will increase the voltage, and therefore the point reading to 60, 70 or even higher. A degenerative process will lower the reading. A chronically ill person often has readings of 35-40, signifying some degenerative processes. More than 600 different measurement points for organs, organic parts, and tissue systems have been worked out and made available to the practitioner.

Once the practitioner has ascertained the area or areas of the body that have inflamed or degenerative readings, it is possible, with EAV, to test homeopathic remedies by inserting them into the circuit via a brass plate. This remedy, or medicament, will influence the body's energetic circuit, and changes may be observed in the point readings. There has yet to be a scientific explanation of this phenomenon, but many successful practitioners using this modality know it to be fact. One possible explanation is that the energetic emissions from the remedy on the plate are able to effect some change on the organ or organ meridian being measured. Another explanation may be that the remedy emission matches, in some way, the emission from the organ or meridian.

Whatever the explanation, EAV, if employed by a skilled practitioner or technician, can determine the effectiveness and compatibility of homeopathic remedies. Having ascertained the worst areas, e.g. the liver, lymphatic system, or small intestine, etc., he or she can test low-potency combination remedies or even Mother Tinctures to ascertain which will "clean up" the patient, and begin to aid healing. Using electroacupuncture or Vega to test homeopathic remedies has been called Resonance Homeopathy, by Dr. Helmut Schimmel of Germany (father of the Vega system). He claims that Resonance Homeopathy is "Three to five times more effective than conventional homeopathy."[47]

One can also use this method to diagnose a specific pathogen. For example, Helicobacter Pylori, known to cause stomach ulcers, is available in a nosode. In an infected person, the raised measurement point of stomach or duodenum will return to the normal reading of 50 when this nosode of H. Pylori is placed on the plate. The practitioner, can, in similar fashion, test other pathogens, sarcodes, drainage remedies, and even confirm his choice and potency of constitutional remedy. EAV has proven to be an invaluable diagnostic tool for the practitioner.

Controversy

There has been much controversy around Electrodermal Screening or Vega testing. While I admit there are concerns with regard to reproducibility, practitioner error, etc., I recommend you do not dismiss this modality out of hand. The various "quack watch" sites simply denigrate and mock, without consideration for the damage they may do. For indeed, what damage does EAV do? Even if inconclusive, there is no harm done to the patient, and I have seen remarkable results throughout my career.

As for the argument that this kind of diagnostic procedure prevents the patient receiving orthodox forms of diagnostic tests, I have found that reputable homeopaths across the country try to work with the patient's primary physician, and/or send clients back to their doctors for blood work, ultrasounds, CT scans, etc, for diagnosis. This protects all involved from legal issues, but more importantly, provides a level of caution and all possible information to the clients or patients themselves.

Without diving further into the complex "For" and "Against" arguments in this book, I send those of you who are interested to this site, and an excellent article written by John Morley, MBAcC, MMAA, MSocBiol Med. Hardly a slouch or charlatan, John held several degrees in acupuncture and Chinese Medicine, and in his lifelong study and practice, helped thousands of people by the use of natural modalities. For more, read this concise and articulate: "Controversy surrounding the Vegatest and Electrodermal Screening

Another helpful article is: "Biological Medicine" by Dr Robert Jacobs, MRCS, LRCP.
http://www.wholisticresearch.com/info/artshow.php3?artid=8
1

Complex Homeopathy

If an electrodermal screening method such as EAV or Vega is not used, success can certainly be achieved through various other means. As stated previously, a classical homeopath would take the case, and prescribe one single remedy which most closely matches all the symptoms and characteristics of the patient. Although this can be very successful, an easier way to ensure some movement in the right direction with regard to symptoms would be to choose two or three drainage and detoxification combinations to drain and support the organs and reduce symptoms. For example, one could use BHI/Heel's excellent combination remedies, and without benefit of Voll testing I would perhaps choose Gallium Heel, Aletris, and Engystol, depending on the symptoms presented. (These would be for a suspected viral involvement.) Of course, a combination of viral nosodes makes this cocktail more powerful. (See the section on Nosode treatment for more information).

Lymphomyosot is also extremely useful, a Heel combination from Germany which includes low potencies of Geranium, Nasturtium, Ferrum Jodatum, Juglans Regia,

Myosotis, Scrophularia, Teucrium, Equisetum, Pinus Sylvestris, Sarsaparilla, Calcium Phosphoricum, and Thyroidinum. These remedies help to drain and support the detoxification of the lymphatic system, skin, liver, and kidneys.

Although there are many who still are adamant that only one remedy is employed at a time, research is showing that combinations of remedies in low-potency work very well indeed.[48] [49] Good results are being obtained by employing several low-potency or MT remedies at the same time. An example of this technique is to use Mother Tinctures or low potencies of Cantharis, Equisetum, Solidago, and Berberis for renal support and drainage, taking great care that the patient does not take too much, or for too long. This way one gains symptom relief quickly. Mother Tinctures are, in actual fact, acting on the herbal plane, and herbalists teach that combinations of herbs are even more effective than single herbs, following the axiom, "The whole is greater than the sum of the parts."

This I have certainly found to be true even with low-potency combinations (1x – 3x) for drainage and organ support. This is being used with great regularity in Germany and France, and to a lesser extent in the UK and the US. Dr. Helmut Schimmel states, "to the best of my knowledge, about 50% of general practitioners and internists also practice Functional Medicine to some extent."[50] Functional Medicine is Dr. Schimmel's term for the system of medicine which employs bioenergetic testing (Voll and Vega), homeopathic single remedies, complexes, nosodes, sarcodes, etc.

Phases Of Illness

According to Dr. Reckeweg, noted German homotoxicologist, illness is the body's attempt to free itself of exogenous and endogenous toxins. If it fails in this attempt, the toxins are driven deeper into the body. According to the six-phase list below, this means to the bottom of the list. The illness progresses in phases, eventually crossing the biological division and entering the cellular phases.

(For more info, see: http://www.vitalitylink.com/article-homeopathy-692-hans-heinrich-reckeweg-father-homotoxicology-heel)

It helps to understand these phases of illness, when deciding how to progress with a weak patient. According to Dr. Reckeweg's table, disease tends to progress in the following phases:

- Excretion phase

- Reaction phase

- Deposition phase

- Impregnation phase

- Degeneration phase

- Neoplasm phase [51]

The excretion phase refers to the ability of the body to dispose of an invading organism through its excretory organs of lungs, kidneys, skin, and bowel (feces). The reaction phase signifies the fight that the immune system of the body engineers against the organism. This would include symptoms such as inflammatory sinus drainage, vaginal discharge, etc. The deposition phase involves storing the toxins within the mesenchyme or Matrix (connective tissue), signaling the beginnings of failure of the body to fight off the invader. This is a sign that the immune system response was unsuccessful.

However, these first three phases do not touch the chemical composition of the cell, and do not influence its structure. Once the deposition and impregnation phases have been reached the body is trying to adapt, to live with, the disease. This is the stage at which homeopathy and homotoxicology are most effective in "re-arousing" the organism to reactivity.

The last three phases are made up of processes that lead to damage, transformation, and eventual destruction of the cell. Reckeweg refers to these latter phases as "cellular phases" as compared to the first three which he termed "humoral phases." Phase 4 (Impregnation) includes toxic damage to cells and cytoplasmic structures. Phase 5

(Degeneration) signals even deeper damage, to essential enzyme systems, such as those of the Krebs cycle, the mitochondria, etc. Phase 6 (Neoplasm) includes damage to the DNA and RNA, and tumor formation.

It is important for the practitioner to plot the course of treatment for a patient with Chronic Fatigue Syndrome based on an awareness of the patient's current phase of illness. The case history, Voll testing results, and the reaction to the first drainage remedies prescribed, will help to determine this. In degeneration stages (the last three phases) the vital force has little energy with which to fight, and one must take care not to prescribe remedies that further weaken the body.

Chronic Fatigue Syndrome is a syndrome in which the body has been unable to successfully throw off toxins. There is a disturbed and sometimes over-active immune system that is causing inflammation, characterized by the symptoms of aches and pains that the CFS patient reports, along with the fatigue, the swollen lymph nodes, and general feelings of being unwell. The liver is overburdened, and therefore the toxins that should be cleared are carried by the blood, where they eventually are deposited (deposition phase) into connective and fatty tissue, such as muscles and joints, and even into the brain, where inflammation occurs. The goals of treatment are to stimulate oxidative metabolism, open detoxification pathways, regulate and cleanse the disturbed immune system, find and treat old foci and old toxins, and to provide supportive treatment for symptoms until the above measures take effect.

After initial drainage and nosode work has been accomplished, it is important to continue to test the patient. In a patient who is still in reaction phase, the vital force (hand to hand reading) will be 85, or will even register inflammation, i.e. 95. These patients tend to recover the most quickly. This is due to the fact that for these people the prescribed remedies simply help the body in the fight it is already generating. The CFS victims that recover more slowly are those who are in later phases, either impregnation or degeneration. This invariably means a lowered vital force reading.

It is interesting to note, in these cases, that after administration of several weeks of low-potency drainage, nosodes, and organ therapy remedies, the vital force will become higher, often even rising to an inflammation state, signifying a move to the reaction phase. This is very rewarding, and one can encourage the patient, who can see the vital force reading improve, even though at this point they perhaps do not feel dramatically better. One can explain to him that now the body is once again fighting, and he will soon see and feel improvement.

Viral or Bacterial Nosode Treatment

If one has employed a Voll, Vega or even Kinesiological screening, a viral match may be found, the most common in CFS being Cytomegalovirus, Coxsackie B1-B6 (B influenza), Mononucleosis (Glandular fever), Human Herpes virus Type 6 (HHV6), or Epstein Barr. Or if digestive issues are paramount, H Pylori may match. It is also possible that one of the "Bowel Nosodes" may match, and be chosen as part of the treatment. (See the section on Bowel Nosodes).

Let me stop here for a moment and define nosode, probably a new term to you. A nosode (from nosos, the Greek word meaning disease) is a homeopathic remedy made from diseased or pathological products such as respiratory discharges, blood, fecal, urinary, or diseased tissue or pus from an infection. It may sound awful, but the remedy, once diluted repeatedly with alcohol and water, is powerful in its ability to cure, yet harmless in terms of pathology.

If a virus or bacteria is suspected, or is diagnostically proven, a nosode should be prescribed. A common method is to take one dose of 30c of the nosode remedy every three days for three weeks. The understanding of past homeopathic practitioners has been to employ the 30c potency of nosodes only once in 6 months, but in my experience, this is simply not enough. I began my practice in this manner, and found that the patient returned in two to three weeks testing just as strongly for the virus. Yet when he took the remedy at frequent intervals for several weeks, the symptoms, and the test match disappeared in three to four weeks.

It is always possible that one may have to instruct the patient to take a short break in this treatment, to allow some intermediary detoxification to take place. There have been many occasions where a 200c of the nosode tested, possibly indicating that the person has harbored the virus, or the viral memory, for a longer period of time. In this case a dose once a week for three weeks has been effective, with doses of the 30c potency, as well, every two to three days, depending on the level of illness of the patient and his or her sensitivity to remedies. If a client/patient is extremely sensitive, it is wise to remember the "Less is more!" mantra, and leave time in between doses.

It is often the case that it is simply impossible to ascertain whether a virus is involved in the CFS patient's ill health. Or if a virus is suspected, which one could it be? There is little to be lost by trying a shotgun treatment: a combo of viruses that are most apt to be involved. For example, Reckeweg sells a wonderful viral combo remedy simply called R88, and I often started a patient on this remedy. It included flu nosodes, Coxsackie, Epstein Barr, Cytomegalovirus, Herpes Simplex and others. American readers can obtain R88 at this website: www.EmporiumOnNet. Those of you from the United Kingdom can find it here: www.EmporiumOnNet.co.uk. There are other viral homeopathic combos available that are worth a try such as www.DesBio Virus Plus. However, I have no personal experience of these others, but you may find it hard to get R88.

(Also please note that some nosodes require prescriptions, so you may have to ask your medical doctor for help.)

If there is improvement after three weeks on R88 (and two or three weeks after this to rest and review), then it is time to use a 30c of an individual nosode, as per the instructions above. Which one, you ask? If you have no means to diagnose, try the R88 ingredients, in nosode form, one at a time. Yes, this may be time-consuming, but so are years and years of CFS/M.E. But I would start with Coxsackie B4, then Epstein Barr, then Cytomegalovirus.

See Ainsworths online, in the UK:
http://www.ainsworths.com/index.php?node=_RemedyStore2 &.

It is essential, as well, during this nosode therapy, to employ drainage support, as described above. Without it, the patient can experience a severe aggravation of his symptoms. If the patient is severely compromised and weak, it is a good idea to prescribe the drainage remedies for approximately a week or even longer, with Vitamin C and lots of pure water, before taking of the first dose of the nosode remedy. In these weakened individuals, it is definitely safer and easier on the patient to start with a 30c of the nosode, even though the 200c may test.

Often, at this time, a single constitutional remedy will test, or be chosen according to standard homeopathic practice. If this is the case, one can also prescribe a 30c to be taken every other day, with the proviso that the vital force is strong enough (at least 80 on the Dermatron/RM10 Voll machine.) If the vital force is weakened, even this middle potency can cause an aggravation, an undesirable reaction in a compromised individual. If there is any doubt, it is preferable to wait until gentle drainage and nosode work has been completed, sometimes as little as three to four weeks, but often longer. Each patient is different, and will recover at a different speed. A patient whose vital force is depleted, (hand-to-hand reading is well below the ideal 84) is in a deeper, more chronic, and more pathological phase of disease.

Bowel Nosodes

The bowel nosodes are a group of remedies prepared from cultures of non-lactose fermenting flora of the intestinal tract. They were studied and brought to our attention by Dr. Edward Bach in 1926 and later expanded upon by Dr. John Paterson and his wife, Elizabeth. Through Bach's and the Patersons' research and clinical studies, they concluded that certain intestinal pathogens have a strong connection to many chronic diseases. [52]

Although the nosodes are less well known than other homeopathic remedies, this is changing, in great part because of our growing awareness of the problems of food allergies, leaky gut issues, and antibiotic damage prevalent in today's patients. [53]

It is important to remember that bowel nosodes are deep acting, and will affect the patient's whole system, not just the digestive tract. They are used one at time, and should only be selected if the well-chosen remedy fails to act or to act and hold. [54]

Candida Albicans and Other Yeasts

Another common problem that may be discovered during testing, and requires nosode treatment, is the intestinal yeast Monilia Albicans, Candida Albicans, or Candida Parapsilosis. Overpopulation of yeast is often involved in the CFS picture. Alternate practitioners, and even physicians who bridge the gap between conventional and alternate medicines, are beginning to accept the validity of this infection. Various clinicians, such as Dr. William Crook, who wrote *Chronic Fatigue Syndrome and the Yeast Connection*, and Dr. Jesse Stoff, who wrote *Chronic Fatigue Syndrome: The Hidden Epidemic*, have repeatedly warned of the part Candida has to play. It must be ruled out before diagnosing CFS, according to Dr. Stoff. Dr. Crook speculates that this yeast overpopulation of the bowel, due to antibiotic use and poor diet of sugars and processed foods, can create a precursor situation for Chronic Fatigue Syndrome.

Some of the symptoms of systemic Candida overgrowth resemble those of CFS, and it is routinely accepted, by alternate practitioners of all types, that this must be ruled out before the diagnosis of CFS can be made. Recurrent yeast infections, fatigue, foggy thinking, disturbed digestion, bloating, gas, intermittent diarrhea and constipation, and itching, are some of the symptoms of this yeast overgrowth of the bowel.

As a natural constituent of the colon, Candida will always be present to some extent. When it moves out of balance, creating a situation known as dysbiosis of the bowel flora, problems can begin. Normally Candida Albicans exists as a relatively harmless component of the intestinal flora. However, if conditions in the bowel are out of balance, it can turn into a troubling invasive form (mycelial form). It sends out root-like shoots, which can penetrate the intestinal mucosa. Unfortunately, given our Western life-style, the conditions are often "right" for this change to occur. Diet plays an important part, as yeast grows rapidly on simple carbohydrates, like refined white sugar. Other factors contribute to the atmosphere that encourages Candida overgrowth, such as low fiber diets, poor digestive function such as achlorhydria, (lack of hydrochloric acid), recurrent use of antibiotics, steroids, the birth control pill, and even chronic stress.

The average human being can tolerate a certain load of Candida in the intestines. However, a series of events such as stress, illness, poor diet, etc., can lead to chronic problems such as impaired immunity, disruption of normal body flora and chemistry, altered acid/alkaline balance, and possible terrain ripe for further infection.

Although it is true that some practitioners are claiming that Candida overgrowth may be the cause of CFS, in fact it is more of an opportunistic infection rather than the main source of the illness. And, unfortunately, it is also true that there are practitioners who seem to be on a "Candida Bandwagon," seeing Candida in everyone they meet. I personally have tested Candida in many of the chronically ill patients in my practice, whether they have been diagnosed with CFS or not. It is very prevalent today.

The treatment of Candida overgrowth in the CFS patients is best achieved with the use of a nosode of Candida, 30c, or one or two doses of 200c to begin with, then 30c every other day for several weeks. In addition, often a low-potency of Borax, such as a 6x or 12x, to be taken for a few days at onset of treatment, will help the body fight the fungus/yeast overgrowth. Borax has many of the symptoms of fungal infection; perhaps this explains its helpfulness in these cases, such as gastro-intestinal irritation and diarrhea, apthous ulceration of mucus membranes, distention after eating, white leukorrhea, pruritis of vulva, moldy smelling breath, and itching skin. The classic symptom of "worse for downward movement" does not necessarily apply, but I find Borax often tests, and helps in the case.

It is also important to add to the prescription anti-Candida nutrients and herbs such as Pau D'Arco, capryllic acid, garlic, and acidophilus supplementation to replace the beneficial bacteria to the colon. It is also essential to stress the strong adherence to a sugar-free, alcohol-free diet.

If the Candida infection does not easily clear over several weeks of nosode treatment, drainage remedies, and attention to diet (sugar/alcohol intake, etc.), one must search for a further underlying problem. When Candida will not clear, there may be yet another *focus* underneath, be it parasite, mercury, infection in a root canal, etc., that stops any improvement from "holding." If there remains a problem that is not addressed in the body, i.e. a focus, one will see improvement, but the symptoms will keep returning. (And remember to consider the Bowel Nosodes, described above.)

Focus

As well as a viral involvement, or Candida overgrowth, there may be another factor, or more than one factor, found to be causing ill health in the patient with Chronic Fatigue

Syndrome. This kind of problem is often referred to as a focus (plural is foci). A focus is an area of pathogenic activity or mesenchymal blockage (scar tissue) that is usually not self-limiting, may be active or inactive, symptomatic or a-symptomatic, and influences in some way the processes of the entire body.[55]

CFS is mostly a multi-factorial disorder, with layers of several foci that need to be peeled away. Dr. Helmut Schimmel, the father of Vega testing, states, in his remarkable book, *Functional Medicine*, "The therapy needed is comparable to an archeological digging, layer by layer.... Symptoms develop from the impact of not just a single one, but of several foci." [56]

These foci may be discovered during the Voll or Vega electroacupuncture testing, or as a result of other routine exams, such as blood tests, dental x-rays, stool tests for parasites, etc. The focus may or may not be symptomatic, which can make detection and diagnosis more difficult. A focus is primarily found to be in the head or in the abdomen. Dr. Schimmel believes that 80% of foci are in the head, 15% in the abdomen, and 5% are scars and scar tissue.[57]

Dr Frank Billings, head of the Department of Medicine at the University of Chicago, wrote, in 1914, "Focal infection is most commonly situated in the head, but may be located in any organ or tissue."[58] Eventually he went on to believe that up to 99% of all foci originate in the tonsils or teeth, with the other one per cent arising from other areas, such as sinuses, lungs, and intestines. Suffice it to say that without addressing these foci, homeopathic treatment can be less effective, ineffective, or only temporarily effective.

There exists equipment to perform a "quadrant test" to try to ascertain the area of the body which harbors a focus. The Biotron, made by Andi Electronics in Denmark, feeds a small electrical current through the patient and measures his conductivity via two brass probes. Normal readings are 80-85, while readings which are too low or too high signify a focus. When a reading is too high (above 50) this indicates inflammation, showing that the body is still putting up a fight. Too low a conductivity reading means degeneration, showing that the patient is no longer reacting to the stimulus of the focus. This valuable piece of equipment gives the practitioner a quick, non-invasive, easy way to locate the area of focus in the body; right side of head, left side of head, right side of abdomen, or left side of abdomen. This can also be achieved with any EAV machine such as the RM10, Dermatron, Mora, or with Vega testing, if however slightly less quick and elegant. Even more sophisticated is an S.E.G test (Segmental Electrograph), which is a computerized test of many parts of the body to disclose the specific area of focus, be it right upper abdomen, left lower abdomen, left leg, etc.

Head Foci

Mercury fillings

First, let us consider head foci. These may prove to be in the sinuses, tonsils, teeth or jaw. Foci of the tonsils often are not symptomatic, although the patient may have recurrent sore throats. Homeopathic treatment, with supportive nutrient and herbal therapy, rather than tonsillectomy, is the correct procedure, or at least should be the first line of action. Leaking silver fillings, which are made up of approximately 52% mercury, can be a source or focus. Although the dental community has tried to defend its use of mercury in silver fillings during the recent public debates as to its safety, evidence is extremely strong that mercury fillings *do* leach mercury.[59] [60] 12,000 papers have been published on the dangers of mercury, and more than a few dentists in America have lost their licenses for daring to suggest this out loud. The World Health Organization reviewed the scientific literature on mercury toxicity, and stated that the human retained daily intake from dental amalgams is 3 to 17 mcg of mercury, more than from any possible food source. WHO also concluded that no exposure to mercury vapor, however slight, is harmless.[61] And several European countries, such as Sweden, have taken steps to ban the use of mercury in fillings.

Mercury poisoning can explain a patient's chronic fatigue, due to the fact that mercury interferes with the oxygen carrying capability of red blood cells. It also upsets the bacterial balance in the gut, leading to dysbiosis, or flora imbalance, in the colon. The presence of mercury creates a change in the makeup of the beneficial bacteria that reside in the colon, rendering them incapable of controlling the growth of Candida. This altered bacteria also reabsorbs mercury vapor from the fillings in the mouth, creating an ever-worsening downhill slide. Protein metabolism is affected, and eventually food products go undigested. This can lead to allergy reactions. According to one of the main researchers into dental amalgams, Dr. Murray Vimy, at the University of Calgary in Canada, mercury may be primarily responsible for the proliferation of allergies and Candida overgrowth experienced by adults in their middle years.[62]

The treatment of mercury toxicity needs several fronts. Homeopathically, one can use a potency chord (homaccord) combination of Mercurius, in various potencies from 6x to 30x, with additional drainage remedies (Berberis, Solidago, Equisetum, 3x-6x) to support the kidneys, as they are the main detoxifying organs for mercury. However, it is also possible to use chelation therapy, and/or nutrients to chelate to the mercury and remove it from the body. These are amino acids, calcium and magnesium, selenium, and chlorella. The old fillings need to be replaced with white composite fillings, but only by a dentist trained in the correct protocol, which serves to protect the patient from further injury by the drilling of the mercury. This protocol includes the removal of the fillings in the correct order, decided by taking galvanic readings, using a rubber dam in the mouth, and nasal oxygen therapy during the dental work. If the patient cannot undergo the removal of the fillings, either due to severe health, or financial considerations, it is possible to improve their health somewhat and maintain them until this work can be done. If mercury toxicity is one of the major underlying causes of the patient's chronic fatigue, it is unlikely a true recovery can be made without the removal of the offending fillings.

Root Canals

Root canalled teeth are also proving to be the source of many health problems, but one hears little about it from dentists, rather from practitioners in the alternate and complementary health field. It is indeed true that here in America dentists are in great danger of having their licenses revoked by the dental board in their state for suggesting that root canalled teeth be pulled, or for even suggesting that mercury fillings be replaced. But, a vast amount of research has recently come to light that brings up questions about the safety of the root canal procedure.

Dr. Weston Price, director of research at the American Dental Association for 14 years, published many articles with regard to his 25 years of research into the dangers of root canals. Although these articles were published back in the 1920s, his work has been compiled and published again by one of the founding member of the American Association of Endodontists, Dr. George Meinig. This excellent book is entitled *Root Canal Cover-Up*.

The research shows how bacteria become trapped in the tubules of the root-canalled tooth. The tooth is dead, its nerve removed, and this lifeless area can put up no immune response to eradicate the problem. Even antibiotics cannot reach into these tubules, which become a source of infection for the entire body. Dr. Price's research clearly shows that systemic illnesses can occur following root canal procedures.

One can also find a connection between more specific, localized pain, and a problem root canalled tooth. It is helpful to utilize the standard teeth-to-organ chart, which shows the connection between specific teeth and a corresponding organ, according to acupuncture meridians. For example, a recent patient of mine gained a dramatic improvement in shoulder and arm pain and stiffness when she had a root-canalled premolar pulled. The effect was instant, she recalled. Five hours after the extraction she noticed all the pain had disappeared. It is useful to bear this in mind with CFS patients who have so many muscle and joint pains.

Voll testing can also detect a root canal problem in the teeth, and one can use the German Staufen nosodes to ascertain bacterial focus. These are Ostitis, Pulpitis, Root Canal TX, Pulpitis (chronic), Ostitis (exudative), Ostitis of the jaw, and Corynebacterium Anaerobe. These are best used diagnostically to determine a problem tooth, as treatment with these nosodes is only of temporary benefit to the patient. The removal of the root-canalled tooth is, unfortunately, the only solution, and it is hard to know how involved the tooth may be in the course of the patient's illness.

However, many patients decide to have a questionable tooth removed, as the level of their suffering demands. It seems worth the gamble, to try to regain their health. In my practice I certainly work on many other areas of problems for the person, and try many remedies before suggesting they think about tooth extraction. It is a hard decision, especially when one considers the stance our orthodox dental profession takes with regard to root canals. It, in public at least, loudly voices its confidence in the root canal procedure, and scoffs at any questions that the alternate community, and even the reputable Dr. Meinig, has raised.

Other Head Foci

Sinus infections and allergies to dental metals: Chronic sinus infections can test as a focus in the CFS patient, and must be addressed. This can be done with a nosode of bacteria, such as Peptostreptococcus (available from the German Staufen Company), Pneumococcus, Staphylococcus, Streptococcus Haemolyticus or Viridans, etc. A sarcode of sinus is useful, but the immediate or eventual use of constitutional and/or miasmatic remedies will be imperative to clear the underlying tendency to sinus infections and/or polyps. This is especially true if the sinus focus seems to be the prevailing cause of illness. This may be hard to determine as so many other foci or pathogens seem to be involved in the CFS picture. One must simply find the presenting (or testing) focus and treat it.

Another potential cause of focus, according to Dr. Reinhold Voll, is the dental materials that make up bridges, posts, dentures, etc. These can induce allergies, and unresolved gingivitis can sometimes be the result, along with a potential for further allergic response to other substances.

Abdominal foci

There are several potential focis in the abdomen, such as diverticulitis, chronic appendicitis, oophoritis and ovarian cysts, chronic cholecystitis, hepatitis, or scars from operations, which can set up fields of focus. These can all be tested with routine orthodox diagnostic procedures, or with Staufen or Vega nosodes using electroacupuncture testing. Chronic appendicitis can be difficult to diagnose, and can often be concurrent with dysbiosis, latent colitis, enteritis, or with amoebic infections. Chronic cholecystitis can often present as migraine especially at the crown of the head, and depression, without any direct severe symptomatology in the area of the gall bladder. But the most common abdominal focus in CFS is the parasite, such as Entamoeba Histolytica, and Giardia Lamblia.

Parasites

With digestive disturbances a significant marker in Chronic Fatigue Syndrome, one must search for the cause. As discussed above, digestion can be severely affected by the overgrowth of Candida, but another possibility is the presence of parasites. Giardia Lamblia, Entamoeba Histolytica, and Ascaris, among others, have been found in a high percentage of CFS patients, and may even be at the center of the onion for some CFS patients.

Two renowned parasitologists, Dr. Hermann Bueno and Dr. Leo Galland, conducted a study entitled "Intestinal Protozoa as a Cause of Chronic Systemic Illness." 403 patients with chronic illness similar to Chronic Fatigue Syndrome were tested for parasites, and fully 93% showed protozoa lodged in the intestines. Entamoeba Histolytica appeared in 257 of the patients, making it the main invading organism, with Giardia Lamblia the primary invader in the other 237 patients. Whether the parasite is the instigating factor in the person's decline in health, or simply an opportunist that invades a weakened system, is not known.[63]

Parasitic infections are simply not well addressed by the orthodox establishment, who receive little to no training in how to recognize the symptoms of parasites, or indeed even to consider them as a possibility with regard to chronic illness. They assume that these organisms and worms do not threaten us in our "clean" Western societies.

In the early 90s, parasitologist Dr. Louis Parrish of New York City conducted research to show an astounding incidence of parasitic infection, backed by the US Department of Public Health figures: 25% of the New York City population was then infected with protozoa such as Entamoeba Histolytica, Giardia Lamblia, Blastocystis Hominis, and Dientamoba Fragilis. Current figures are similar: in recent years, CDC reports that approximately 15-25 % of the US population is infected by one or more of Toxocara, Giardia, Entamoeba, Tapeworm, Trichomonas, etc. The CDC surveillance estimate for 2011-2012 is approximately 7% of the US population infected with Giardia, alone.

With digestive disturbances a significant marker in Chronic Fatigue Syndrome, one must search for the cause. As discussed above, digestion can be severely affected by the overgrowth of Candida, but another possibility is the presence of parasites. Giardia Lamblia, Entamoeba Histolytica, and Ascaris, among others, have been found in a high percentage of CFS patients, and may even be at the center of the onion for some CFS patients.

Therefore, as much as we may be brought up to believe our food and water are clean, and these types of issues only occur in the undeveloped countries, this is simply not the case. Parasitic infection is on the rise, perhaps due to foreign wars, the increase of international travel, and untrained immigrant food handlers.

The actual symptoms of protozoa infection mimic those of Chronic Fatigue Syndrome to a great extent. Morton Walker, medical journalist and co-author *of The Downhill Syndrome*, with Dr. Pavel Yutsis, theorizes that parasite invasion and infection is one of the main trigger of Chronic Fatigue Syndrome.[64] Protozoa infection causes persistent tiredness, excessive yet unrefreshing sleep, gastrointestinal symptoms such as malabsorption, acid reflux, gas, mucous in the stools, irritable bowel syndrome (intermittent diarrhea and constipation), a general feeling of being unwell, or sensations of toxicity. These include lack of concentration, confused memory, nightmares, musculo-skeletal pains, wide swings in blood sugar, and menstrual irregularities.[65] All of these reported symptoms occur frequently in those diagnosed with Chronic Fatigue Syndrome.

Parasites, including Entamoeba Histolytica, Giardia, and others, can literally puncture the digestive tract, allowing macromolecules of undigested foods into the blood stream, where the immune system begins to attack them as foreign invaders. Not only does this lead to allergenic overload, but also to nutritional deficiency and toxicity.[66] The immune system literally has to try to finish up the digestion process, leading to an up-regulation of the immune system, with the inherent inflammation and allergic state that this entails.

Although parasitologist and researchers have discovered a large percentage of CFS sufferers with parasites, especially Giardia Lamblia, Entamoeba Histolytica, and Ascaris, this does not necessarily mean they are the initiating factor in the syndrome. It is just as possible that due to the immune altering processes of this illness, and the undisputed intestinal involvement, that the patient becomes *more vulnerable* to parasites taking hold, whereas they would be fought off in a strong and healthy person. An example of this is the fact that in studies of AIDS victims has shown that virtually every AIDS patient is infected with amebiasis or giardiasis.[67] This of course does not prove a causal relationship. The complexities of Chronic Fatigue Syndrome, such as they are, mean that we still just don't know exactly how this illness comes about in various individuals. A great many CFS victims do prove to have parasites, and the treating of this problem does lead to improvement, but there are those who don't. In that case, the practitioner must ascertain whether other toxic agents or foci are actively involved.

To compound the problem, Voll and Vega testing sometimes does not adequately test these parasites – perhaps they send out blocking frequencies. It is true that many parasites are masters of fooling the body into thinking nothing is wrong, and perhaps this affects our Voll readings. Therefore, it is vital that one always do purged stool tests if one suspects parasites at all, and even then not trust a negative test. Dr. Omar Amin of the Institute of Parasitic Diseases in Arizona states that one must see four consecutive negative purged stool tests before one can trust a parasite has been eradicated. Dr. Louis Parrish agrees. Discussing stool specimens, he states, "If they are negative and one is clinically suspicious, get three to six more."[68] Knowing how difficult it can be to detect parasites in the stool leads us to doubt the results of a single non-purged stool test, as requested by the standard MD for a patient suffering from diarrhea after a trip to Mexico or Thailand.

Therefore, if in doubt regarding the presence of parasites, it is wise to conduct several purged stool tests, or even try a diagnostic course of anti-parasitic herbs and homeopathic remedies to see if some improvement is achieved, even if the Voll, Vega, or Kinesiology testing is negative or inadequate. The homeopathic remedies useful in this endeavor, or for proper treatment of a discovered parasitic infection, are Artemisia Vulgaris, Tanacetum Vulgare, Filix Mas, Absinthium, Cina, Chenopodium Anthelminticum, Mercurius Corrosivus, Ascaris Nosode, Ameba Nosode, Filarinose Nosode, Oxyuren nosodes, Taenia nosode, Trichinose nosode, and other nosodes of specific suspected or diagnosed parasites.

Having discovered a parasite in the patient with Chronic Fatigue Syndrome, treating with the nosode of the individual parasite is very effective, such as recommending 30c of the appropriate nosode every other day for three weeks. It is also important to back up this treatment with the herbal extracts of Wormwood, Black Walnut Hull Tincture, Quassia, Garlic, Grapefruit Seed, Olive Leaf, and cloves. Fiber and herb combinations aimed at gently scraping clean the intestinal walls are also very helpful, plus soothing herbs such as marshmallow root and slippery elm help to calm the inflamed tissues of the digestive tract.

Treatment of Allergies

Clinical ecologists and other practitioners have full time jobs allergy testing and giving desensitization injections, which routinely take several years of weekly shots. And they are not guaranteed to be effective for the allergic sufferer. However, desensitizing, using specific allergens in homeopathic dilutions can be even more effective, cheaper and painless. One must certainly address why the body became hyper-reactive, i.e. allergic, in the first place, whether due to chronic overload of stress, heavy metals, infections, or to miasmatic influences. But, initially, to desensitize regularly eaten foods, or something as prevalent and pervasive as sinus allergies to dust, or pollens, can be a blessing to the patient, while deeper work is carried out. Since a very high proportion of CFS patients suffer from allergies, it is vital to take this into consideration in the treatment plan.

If the practitioner decides to use low potencies to desensitize the specific allergen, great care must be taken in administration. Many of these substances are available as over-the-counter bottles of homeopathic combinations, such as "Mold/Yeast/Dust" or "Animal Dander," or "Grass Pollens." The recommended dose on most of these bottles is ten drops three times a day, but for many allergic individuals, especially those with Chronic Fatigue Syndrome, this can be too much. Sometimes *way* too much. It is wise and prudent to advise the patient to take two drops once a day for two days, then twice a day for two days. Then she can continue to add a drop each day so that the dose builds up to ten drops three times a day in this manner. It is not unusual for someone to take six weeks to be able to handle 5 or 6 drops of the homeopathic allergen. But this kind of treatment tends to shave the edge off the hypersensitivity of the patient, making her less reactive. There is often a substantial reduction in symptoms using this method, especially if there is no underlying focus to be resolved.

Allergy reactions and symptoms seem to work along the lines of "the cup runneth over." There only seems to be so much the sensitive person can take, before allergies develop. It starts often with just one thing, e.g. dust, pollen, dairy, or wheat. But, allergies tend to worsen, to "spread," to multiply, somehow, especially when an unresolved focus or a miasmatic influence is in place. If one is able to desensitize one or two main allergens for the patient, they begin to feel much better, and are somehow less reactive to other allergens.

This, of course, is always best done alongside the course of deeper homeopathic treatment with the constitutional remedy, as it is true that the improvement will often not last or "hold" if allergy desensitization takes place without deeper issues being addressed. In the case of miasmatic allergy, or for those for whom there is no focus, allergies will abate with the correct prescription of the constitutional remedy.

Heavy Metal Toxicity

Mercury toxicity has been addressed above, in the section discussing head foci, and mercury leakage from silver/mercury fillings. But, if any heavy metal is discovered, whether through Voll testing, hair mineral analysis, or blood tests (ideally following a DMPS provocation), the eradication of the metal will help enormously in the movement of the patient towards health.

Although EAV is unable to give the practitioner actual levels in the body, it will certainly indicate the presence of lead, aluminum, cadmium, etc. A hair mineral analysis is also useful, both before and after treatment, to verify the treatment is working.

Using low homeopathic potencies of the offending metal, be it aluminum, mercury, lead, etc., with adequate drainage remedies, will help the body detoxify. For example Mercurius 6x, Alumina 6x, or Plumbum 6x can be employed to reduce the load of the heavy metal in the body. The source of the metal must be found and eliminated, whether it is a bridge in the dental work that has nickel, tin, etc., or whether it is cadmium toxicity in a barmaid who breathes cigarette smoke many hours a day.

Other remedies that are known to reduce heavy metal toxicity are listed in the repertory and may be employed if indications match, such as, for lead toxicity, Alumina, Causticum, Tuberculinum, Alumen, Belladonna, Colocynthis, Natrum Sulphuricum, Platina, Sulphur, Terebinthina, and Veratrum Album. Mercury toxicity can be addressed with Aurum Metallicum, Carbo Vegetabilis, Kai Iodatum, Lachesis, Mercurius, Phytolacca, Natrum Sulphuricum, Staphisagria, Sulphur, Nitricum Acidum, and others. Several remedies listed for aluminum poisoning are Alumina, Bryonia, and Plumbum Metallicum.

Chelation therapy is another adjunct therapy to speed this process, as is the use of amino acids, calcium and magnesium, selenium in the case of mercury, and sea vegetables such as Chlorella to help chelate the toxic metal out of the body. This heavy metal toxicity acts as a systemic focus, and certainly has to be addressed before cure will hold in the body.

Sleep Disorders

Disordered sleep is one of the main symptoms of CFS. Although exhausted, the patient reports she simply cannot stay asleep, whether due to aches and pain, a sensation of nervous tension, frequent and stimulating dreams, or from feeling feverish. Of course, these symptoms will be considered in the entire picture of the patient, and may be

addressed with the constitutional remedy. There are indeed
many remedies listed in the repertory under "insomnia"; more
than 30 as three-point remedies, and more than 80 listed as
two point remedies. However, it can be very beneficial to
prescribe a low-potency remedy, or combination of remedies,
to help with sleep, until the detoxification and drainage has
taken place. These are 1x-3x of Valeriana, Avena Sativa,
Passiflora, Chamomilla, and Coffea. In herbal form, Passion
Flower, GABA, Theanine, Valerian, Oats, Poppy, and
occasional Kava can be an alternative.

A gentle antihistamine used as an occasional sleep agent
can be very helpful, such as the effective ingredient in
Benadryl, diphenhydramine. A half a capsule of this drug
occasionally will give the patient a better, if not good night
sleep. However, some patients will experience some heart
racing or mild palpitations if they take it too often. Even an
occasional small dose of dimenhydrinate (such as
Dramamine) will help ensure at least some rest and sleep. I
always suggest these over the counter drugs be saved for
occasional use; in my experience, with the correct use of
homeopathic remedies and herbs, the Chronic Fatigue
sufferer will be improving so much that they do not need to
employ this sort of help for long.

Muscle Pain

If muscle pain is one of the most prominent and disturbing symptoms to the patient, one must take these symptoms and the corresponding modalities into account when choosing remedies for the CFS patient. Arnica, Rhus Toxicodendron, Dulcamara, Rheum, Ruta, to name but a few, are remedies that will be helpful in this regard.

Once again, BHI/Heel makes combination homeopathic remedies that are very useful for this problem. One such remedy, Traumed tablets, (plus Traumed cream) are combinations of the above remedies, plus others that can help this discomfort. I also find that Discus Compositum and Rheuma-Heel are of benefit.

It is also important to check other remedies which may be involved in this muscle discomfort. Brucella, Toxoplasmosis, and Coxsackie B, must be ruled out, or treated if present, as these infectious agents often present with muscle pain. Also, there is some evidence that muscle and joint pain can be a result of a toxic reaction to vaccines, especially the common MMR (Measles /Mumps/ Rubella) vaccine.

Many patients find that ibuprofen helps the muscle pains, but many do not wish to take this drug often due to its ability to cause intestinal disturbance. Also, there is some indication that Ibuprofen and other non-steroidal anti-inflammatory drugs weaken or destroy cartilage (a sad irony for the many people with arthritis that constantly swallow these drugs).[69]

I often suggest an alternative to patients that do seem to obtain relief from ibuprofen; to open an ibuprofen capsule and mix it with a little moisturizing lotion or even with Traumed cream) and rub this right on the trigger point of the muscle where the pain and discomfort occurs. It is amazingly helpful. Once again, I would hope that the correct remedies are being employed to help the patient rid herself of the pain to begin with, to make this use of a drug unnecessary.

Along with the right homeopathic remedies, I have found the New Zealand Green Lipped mussel oil extract is powerful anti-inflammatory, especially for arthritis patients. For those patients with Chronic Fatigue Syndrome who experience predominant muscle and joint aches, this potent Omega 3 oil often brings an anti-inflammatory effect.

CONSTITUTIONAL OR CLASSICAL HOMEOPATHY

It is possible to save the detailed "taking of the case," for the purpose of choosing the constitutional remedy, until several weeks into the case. Of course, the practitioner must learn, in thorough homeopathic manner, every detail of the symptoms and modalities, plus gain a thorough understanding of the characteristics and personality of the patient, in order to find the similimum.

One cannot over emphasize the importance of the constitutional remedy during treatment of the CFS patient. It is possible, even probable, that the remedy choice will change in the progression of treatment, as one peels away up the "onion layers' of the patient's health problems. It is rare that only one remedy would suffice for the CFS patient during the course of treatment.

Later in the treatment, when the CFS patient has improved a great deal, one begins to recognize the remedy that is closely associated with his or her basis nature, such as Calcarea Carbonicum, Sepia, Sulphur, or Natrum Muriaticum. This is in contrast to the beginning of treatment, when one is usually drawn to choose one of the remedies that match the symptoms of Chronic Fatigue Syndrome, of course with the consideration of the modalities, personality, etc., of the patient. However, there are exceptions to this. Some CFS patients, after nosode treatment and drainage, will respond dramatically to their original (possibly) constitutional remedy. Perhaps these are the people who have been ill the least length of time, have strong constitutions, and/or have fewer layers to their illness.

After the first prescription, very often the symptom picture will change, and one may go through several deep-acting, constitutional remedies before the patient returns to a high level of health. This is always the case in any deep work in the homeopathic modality. Any chronic illness will take time, and there are often several changes of prescription before success is achieved.

In this regard, Chronic Fatigue Syndrome is not unlike any other illness. It is possible that a remedy that matches the CFS symptoms will help the patient greatly, to be followed by a remedy that more closely matches the patient's constitutional symptoms. As a new symptom picture emerges, one follows the homeopathic rules, and chooses a new similimum, when one is sure that a change is required.

Repertorization

So, how does a homeopath decide upon and recommend a certain remedy? In a rather simplistic nutshell, the homeopath "takes the case," which means collecting all pertinent facts about the patient, using history-taking, observation, clinical data, etc., then employs knowledge of the Homeopathic Materia Medica, Organon of Medicine, and the Repertory.

Homeopathy treats the ill person in totality, rather than just focusing on the diseases or conditions they suffer from. Therefore, the practitioner concentrates on the patient's unique experience of their illness, plus all the basic characteristics of her nature, mental state, and physicality. This is in contrast to the orthodox doctor's method: he simply looks at basic symptoms and physical abnormalities in order to prescribe.

Many criteria may play into the homeopath's choice of remedy. Here are a few:

- The patient's history; long term symptoms before current illness

- Parent's history and illnesses

- The current symptoms

- An instigating factor: "never well since _____."

- Totality of the symptoms

- Recurrent symptoms

- Mental state

- General symptoms such as "feels the cold," better in the evening," "craves sweets," etc.

- Specific peculiar symptoms. Examples: a recurrent dream of snakes, a sensation that the brain is swollen, cold knees at night, a headache that is always on the right side in a specific spot, etc.

Armed with all of this information, a homeopath *repertorizes* the case, either by hand or by the use of computer software (more and more common nowadays). Searching for a remedy that covers all of the above criteria, each piece of information is graded according to importance, to its weight in the case. Strong symptoms are considered first, those that are intense, recurrent, peculiar, or expressed spontaneously and clearly. Then the practitioner adds general symptoms, then local, then modalities. The homeopath looks for rubrics (symptoms as written in a homeopathic repertory) that describe the true essence or the essential features of the case, and chooses a single matching remedy that will hopefully instigate the cure and return the patient to health.

Chronic Fatigue Syndrome Remedies

Most of the major repertories, i.e. Clarke, Kent, and Boericke, do not list Chronic Fatigue Syndrome, as this term is fairly new, dating only from the last twenty years or so. A noted current homeopath, Robin Murphy, ND, has written a

modern Repertory, published in 1993, which does list
Chronic Fatigue Syndrome.[70]

The three-point remedies listed under Chronic Fatigue
Syndrome by Dr. Murphy are Alumina, Ammonium
Carbonicum, Caladium, Calcarea Carbonicum, Carcinosin,
China, Conium, Ferrum, Gelsemium, Graphites, Lachesis,
Nux Vomica, Phosphoricum Acidum, Picricum Acidum,
Silica, and Sulphuricum Acidum.

The two-point remedies are Ambra Grisea, Arsenicum
Album and Iodatum, Aurum Metallicum, Baptisia,
Causticum, Chelidonium, China Sulphuricum, Cocculus,
Digitalis, Kali Carbonicum, Kali Phosphoricum,
Laurocerasus, Lycopodium, Manganum, Mercurius, Natrum
Carbonicum, Natrum Muriaticum, Nux Moschata, Opium,
Phosphorus, Psorinum, Senega, Sepia, Stannum, Stramonium,
Sulphur, Thuja, and Valeriana.

Also of great use from Dr. Murphy's repertory is the
rubric "exertion aggravates." Only one 3-point remedy is
listed, which is Silica. The 2-point remedies are Arnica,
Calcarea, Phosphoricum Acidum, and Rhus Toxicodendron.

Also for "CFS from influenza" Dr. Murphy lists (2
points); Carcinosin, Gelsemium, Phosphoricum Acidum,
Silicea, and (1-point), Kali Phosphoricum and Thuja.

For the rubric "CFS from mono," the following remedies
are listed (3 points): Carcinosin, (2-points): Baptisia,

Calcarea, Gelsemium, Mercurius, Phosphoricum Acidum,
and (1-point) Silicea and Thuja.

These remedies are a good place to start in the choice of
a single classical remedy for the patient with CFS. The basic
rules of homeopathy still apply; one must find the similimum
that matches the totality of symptoms, and not attempt to
prescribe solely for a specific illness. One must keep in mind
that many of the broad polycrest remedies will be of great use
during the course of homeopathic treatment, just as in any
other chronic illness.

The homeopathic Materia Medica holds many remedies
that address the major individual symptoms of CFS;
weakness, fatigue exacerbated by exercise, swollen glands
and recurring sore throats, low grade fever, nervous
exhaustion, and muscle aches and pains. The trick is to find
the correct remedies, often presenting in layers, and to
support the patient in a very depressing, exhausting time of
their lives.

Let us consider a few of the most commonly indicated
remedies one by one:

GELSEMIUM: When the chief complaint of a patient is
weakness, one must consider Gelsemium. In advanced cases,
this can even mean paralysis, since the main action is
centered on the nervous system. The weakness and weariness

is both physical and mental, and the patient complains that he is unable to think, and is forgetful and dull.

Therefore, Gelsemium can often be the perfect picture of the CFS patient, with incapacitating fatigue, muscular weakness, dullness, listlessness, and vertigo. The eyelids are heavy and drooping, and the person can barely open them. The head is heavy. There is fatigue after light exercise, and an aversion to mental work. The patient needing Gelsemium may have chills alternating with flushes of heat, and trembling. The face has the true "worn-out" expression. An interesting keynote to Gelsemium, which helps the practitioner with his choice, is that the symptoms may be alleviated by profuse urination. There may also be a chill, which runs up and down the spine.

Comparison remedies for the consideration of the practitioner include Baptisia, Magnesium Phosphoricum, Stannum, Silica, Lycopodium, Phosphoricum Acidum, or Muriatic Acid.

The life of Gelsemium, according to Miller, is 30 days, but is considered by some to be a relatively shallow acting remedy, not a deep constitutional. However, in the case of CFS, it can be very effective, where indications match.

BAPTISIA: Baptisia, like Gelsemium, has symptoms of excessive prostration, sleepy dullness, and even stupor. However, it tends to be better indicated in serious infections,

characterized by a "besotted' or "drunken" appearance. It is
indicated in cases of influenza, with bruised pains, and the
patient, sore all over, complains that the bed is too hard. The
throat is red and inflamed, there is a wild wandering feeling
in the brain, and the patient is restless. His sleep is disturbed
by wild nightmares. He may even report that he feels he is
scattered around the bed. The discharges are offensive. The
action of the remedy is short, only 6-8 days.

Remedies that are similar for consideration include
Bryonia, Gelsemium, Arsenicum, Rhus Toxicodendron,
Muriatic Acid, Opium, and Pyrogenium.

KALI PHOSPHORICUM: Kali Phosphoricum is another
valuable remedy we can turn to in CFS cases. It is extremely
helpful where there is mental and physical exhaustion,
especially after periods of over-exertion and stress. When this
exhaustion is coupled with nervousness, prostration, and
over-stimulation, Kali Phosphoricum must be considered.
There is brain fag (mental fatigue), and irritable restlessness
and anxiety. The patient feels very nervous, lethargic, and
startles easily. There may be headache with an empty, gone
sensation in the stomach, and a burning sensation that runs
along the spine. The eyelids droop, the tongue has a mustard
colored coating, and the breath is offensive. The patient's
temperature may be low, and he complains of feeling cold.
Arthritic pains of arms and legs are better for motion and
warmth, and there may be shortness of breath, even a

tendency to asthma. The patient is markedly worse for excitement or worry, for physical or mental exertion, for eating, if cold, and in the early morning. He or she is better for warmth and rest. Although Kali Phosphoricum is certainly a deep acting remedy (40-50 days), it is often used in CFS for the above symptoms, not solely as a constitutional remedy.

Remedies for comparison include Picricum Acidum, Gelsemium, Zincum, Muriatic Acid, and Sepia.

PHOSPHORICUM ACIDUM: Like Gelsemium, this remedy causes debility, which produces a nervous exhaustion, so it is also often indicated in CFS cases. Mental debility comes first, followed by physical weakness. Therefore, it can be thought of in cases where the patient reports great stress, grief, or mental worry before onset of the illness. According to Boericke, "Whenever the system has been exposed to the ravages of acute disease, grief, loss of vital fluids, we obtain conditions calling for it. The patient is listless, his memory is impaired, he cannot collect his thoughts or find the right word." His head is heavy, and he is confused. There is vertigo, and great aversion to sunlight. Diarrhea is almost invariably present in the person needing Phosphoric Acid. The extremities are weary, with pains in joints and bones. He craves fruit and fruit juices. There is often hair loss, even from the eyebrows and chest. The duration of this remedy is 40 days, and remedies that should

be considered and compared are Muriatic Acid, Picricum
Acidum, Phosphorus, Sepia, and China.

PICRICUM ACIDUM; This remedy is not unlike Kali
Phosphoricum. They both have nervous prostration as a main
feature, with brain fag, and burning along the spine. There is
the same weary, tired feeling, which is aggravated by the
slightest excitement, exertion, or over-work. However, unlike
those needing Kali Phosphoricum, patients who will benefit
from Picric Acid are ameliorated by cold air and cold water.
Other remedies for comparison are Kali Phosphoricum,
Oxalicum Acidum, Gelsemium, Phosphorus, Phosphoric
Acidum, Silicea, and Argent Nitricum.

SILICA: Silica (Silicea) is a deep, long-acting remedy, which
certainly matches many of the essential symptoms of CFS:
great weariness and debility, a wish to lie down, nervous
debility, and exhaustion from hard work. The patient is faint-
hearted, with a "want of grit." He is restless, fidgety, and
startles easily, at the slightest noise. The patient is always
chilly, with inflammation of the glands, and recurrent colds,
flu, and infections. There is constipation from inactivity of
the rectum. There is a great tendency in the Silica patient to
pus formation, such as pimples, abscesses, boils of the gums,
quinsy etc. The skin tends to crack at the corners of the
mouth, and every injury seems to suppurate, and become
infected. There will be defects of bones, hair, and nails, due

to poor metabolism of minerals. The person needing Silica will feel better from warmth, and in wet or humid weather. The patient is worse at the time of the new moon, in the morning, during menses, and when lying down, especially on the left side.

With regard to the rubric, "exertion aggravates," this is a very important symptom of Chronic Fatigue Syndrome, as it is perhaps essential to the diagnosis of CFS. Silica is strongly indicated for this rubric (3 points in Murphy's Repertory).

When considering Silica with Chronic Fatigue Syndrome in mind, one must compare Calcarea Carbonica, Hepar Sulph, Thuja, Mercurius, Kali Carbonicum, Phosphorus, Fluoricum Acidum (especially if warm blooded) and Picricum Acidum. Silica is believed to be a remedy of long duration, 40 –60 days.

CARCINOSIN: Carcinosin is one of the most valuable remedies in Chronic Fatigue Syndrome, where it is indicated. And yet it has been little employed, especially by American homeopaths. This is due, in part, to the fact that it is a "prescription-only" remedy here in the States. Secondly, it doesn't appear often in the early repertories and Materia Medicas. For example, Boericke and Kent do not list Carcinosin. It is, however, listed in a modern repertory, by Dr. Robin Murphy, N.D., as the only three-point remedy under the rubric "CFS from mononucleosis."

Finally, it is a rather hard remedy to "see" in practice, as symptoms of Carcinosin (or Carcinosinum) are very changeable, contrary, and alternating. For example, there may be both aggravation and amelioration from the same stimulus in the listings. Another example is that the patient may be flabby and overweight, or thin and even emaciated. This complexity may be due to the fact that Carcinosin seems to be a mixture of the three miasms, and the symptoms presenting may depend on which miasm is predominant at that time. At the same time, one may see symptoms of a remedy underneath the Carcinosin, such as a polycrest like Natrum Muriaticum, Silica Calcarea, Carbonicum, Lycopodium, etc. for the patient as well. This can make the choice of remedy difficult.

Persons needing Carcinosin are very often passionate, intense people who over-extend themselves on many levels, due to a sense of being unfulfilled. They tend to work too hard, and push their own limits, often leading to health breakdown. This is very often the type of person who is a victim of Chronic Fatigue Syndrome. Underneath the driving force of his or her nature is often someone who will admit to a sensation of loneliness, or feeling of abandonment. They may suppress their anger, as their low self worth and lack of self-confidence will not allow them to express it. On the other hand, some patients may be rebellious, displaying destructive, or anxious, outbursts. They often are averse to talking, are aggravated from conversation.

Like the other remedies useful in CFS, there may be excessive exhaustion, swollen lymph glands, chronicity of their complaints, and constantly changing symptoms. For example, heat and cold may ameliorate or exacerbate symptoms. They are often oversensitive to homeopathic remedies, and mental symptoms may alternate with physical symptoms. There is very often insomnia, and a malaise or depression that the patient himself cannot understand. Constipation is almost uniform in the patient needing Carcinosin, although there may have been a tendency to diarrhea in childhood. In the literature is listed a discoloration of the skin, known as a unique "café-au-lait" complexion, but this is not essential to the correct choice of Carcinosin. There may, however, be many, or new moles, eruptions, freckles, etc. There is often cancer in the family history, or tuberculosis. Patients needing Carcinosin will often be worse in the afternoon, from 1 P.M. until 6 P.M., and ameliorated in the evening. Open air generally ameliorates, but it is important, once again, to remember that these symptoms can be very changeable, even contrary.

Carcinosin is often useful, like the other miasmatic nosodes, when the indicated remedy fails to act or to hold its action. It can act to "open up" the case in order to pave the way for other remedies. This can hold true even where few of the symptoms match the listed indications. For example, using Carcinosin with a patient who was never well following mononucleosis may clear the path for remedies that more correctly match the symptoms.

According to Roger Morrison, M.D., when considering Carcinosin, it is also useful to study Medorrhinum, Tuberculinum, Arsenicum, Sepia, and Phosphorus. R.D. Micklem, who wrote a composite booklet of many practitioners' findings with regard to Carcinosin, advises us to compare Alumina, Calcarea Phosphoricum, Lycopodium, Natrum Muriaticum, Natrum Sulphuricum, Nux Vomica, Opium, Psorinum, Pulsatilla, Staphisagria, Syphilinum, Thuja, and two of the bowel nosodes, Gaertner, and Dys. Co (prepared from B. Dysenteriae).

SCUTELLARIA: A native plant in North America, scutellaira latifolia, (also known as skullcap) is an herb of the mint family, often used to treat disorders of the nervous system, plus other diseases such as hepatitis and general inflammation. Homeopaths have long employed scutellaria in cases of post-influenza nervous exhaustion and weakness. (Remember Kali Phos for these situations, as well.)

AMMONIUM CARBONICUM: Although highly represented in the repertory, with many rubrics across many systems, this remedy remains somewhat elusive and under prescribed. Ammonium Carb. is a deep-acting, anti-psoric, constitutional remedy, which must be considered when the main complaints of the patient are weakness and exhaustion. Roger Morrison describes it well in his "Desktop Guide to Keynotes and Confirmatory Symptoms." He finds it "a very useful remedy in cases with chronic fatigue or cardiac cases with borderline congestive failure, where endurance is the main complaint of the patient." The person may suffer from palpitations, dyspnea, nervous prostration, and brain fag. The mind is dull, and the patient is sluggish with an oppressed feeling in the chest. There is aching in the bones, and there is often hay fever and a nighttime cough (3:00 a.m.)

Constitutionally, the patient may tend to be heavy set or fat, and often unclean in bodily habits. Glands of the neck may be enlarged, menses may be painful, profuse, and begin with bouts of diarrhea. A keynote, which may aid the prescriber in his choice of Ammonium Carbonicum, is the tendency to epistaxis (nosebleed) while washing the face.

Ammonium Carbonicum is a remedy, which has many rubrics in our repertories. This can tend to confuse its picture. But with some symptoms being so similar to those of CFS, it is essential that it be remembered when trying to find the similimum for our patients with this disorder.

Life of the remedy is reported to be 40 days, and remedies for comparison include Muriatic Acid, Lachesis (similar in action, inimical), Sulphur, Graphites, Carbo Vegetabilis, Calcarea Carbonicum, and Capsicum.

OPIUM: Opium's action is primarily on the cerebro-spinal and nervous system, causing brief excitement, then depression and paralysis of function. It lessens the power of concentration and judgment, stimulates the imagination, leading to many pleasant dreams, or alternately, frightful images. Opium causes a sleepy state, even narcolepsy and coma. Stupor, with insensibly, are main indications that would lead one to think of Opium. Although painlessness and dreaminess are considered essential by some for the prescription of this remedy, two states may actually alternate. That is, of course, the lack of pain, somnolence, almost "blissed-out" condition, or conversely, a hurried, intense state of fear and anguish presides. In this way, Opium must be remembered as a great remedy for ailments brought on by shock or fright. It can act like Sulphur and the miasmatic nosodes, when the indicated remedy fails to act or to hold its action. As per Boericke, "Want of susceptibly to remedies though indicated."

Generally, patients needing homeopathic Opium are warm blooded and aggravated by heat. The eyes are heavy and half-closed. There is constipation with no urge, and the stool consists of round, hard, black balls. The stream of urine may be feeble, the respiration slow, and the patient may sleep extremely heavily, waking with a sense of suffocation.

Opium is an interesting drug in several ways. Of course, it is useful in cases of CFS where indications match. However, it is also overlooked as a "case-opener" and a remedy for use after shock. It is an under used remedy, particularly in the United States, where it is not available. However, when it is indicated, it can be dramatically effective. And it must also be remembered in cases where an opiate miasm may be in place due to the persistent use of acetaminophen/codeine products as painkillers for migraine, dysmenorrhea, etc.

The life of homeopathic Opium is relatively short, at seven days. Remedies for comparison are Baptisia, Nux Vomica, Nux Moschata, Alumina, Calcarea Carbonicum, Belladonna, Gelsemium, Morphinum, and Codeinum.

HOMEOPATHIC RESEARCH

There is growing evidence that homeopathy works,[71] regardless of the vitriolic attacks it regularly receives by the orthodox medical establishment and the press.

The very vocal naysayers of homeopathy shout, "There's nothing in them! There is no remaining molecule of the original substance!" No, but there ARE nanoparticles left. (A nanoparticle is one part per billion). Does that sound too small to matter, or to have any effect? Consider this: dogs can smell substances in parts per billion, or even trillion. This is verifiable science and what the legal world calls "Back Letter Law." If animals can detect a substance in such small quantities, why is it inconceivable that the human immune system can detect a substance even in great dilution?

To bring this point home, I quote from an article by Peter Tyson from NPR's NOVA, 2012:

> *"... dogs can detect some odors in parts per trillion. What does that mean in terms we might understand? Well, in her book Inside of a Dog, Alexandra Horowitz, a dog-cognition researcher at Barnard College, writes that while we might notice if our coffee has had a teaspoon of sugar added to it, a dog could detect a teaspoon of sugar in a million gallons of water, or two Olympic-sized*

*pools worth. Another dog scientist likened their
ability to catching a whiff of one rotten apple in two
million barrels.*"[72]

And there are now several pieces of research to confirm
the presence of physical substance – nanoparticles – in high
homeopathic remedies. Employing Transmission Electron
Microscopy (TEM), electron diffraction and chemical
analysis, several studies in 2010, 2012, and 2013 showed the
presence of these physical particles in the form of
nanoparticles of the starting material.[73]

IR Bell and M Koithan, authors of a study published in
BMC Complementary Alternative Medicine in October 2012,
explained it this way:

*"Homeopathic remedies are proposed as source
nanoparticles... and are distinguished from
conventional bulk drugs in structure, morphology,
and functional properties.... This model provides a
foundation for theory-driven research on the role of
nanomaterials in living systems, mechanisms of
homeopathic remedy actions and translational uses
in nanomedicine.*"[74] [75]

Randomized control trials (RCTs)

When it comes to researching illness or conditions with homeopathic remedies, a basic problem comes to light, one that is routinely overlooked or misunderstood by critics of homeopathy: orthodox, conventional medicine regards randomized control trials as the be-all and end-all in judging treatment or modality. The essential issue with RCTs, (randomized control trials) is that they are simply not an appropriate or balanced assessment of evidence, when it comes to homeopathic practice. Observational studies are more useful when it comes to the way homeopathy is practiced.

Why? One substance, as tested in standard research trials, aiming for a cure in every patient, goes against the natural grain of homeopathy. This RCT model of measuring drug or treatment efficacy does not allow for the fact that in homeopathy, practitioners tailor remedy choice very specifically to the individual. The prescription is chosen based on a multitude of factors: personality, family health history, lifestyle, emotional health, likes and dislikes of the patient, even whether he or she is warm-blooded or cold-blooded. Therefore, how well a chosen remedy works for a patient is extremely hard to quantify with a randomized control trial.

But, even accepting that RCTs do not adequately or fairly judge homeopathic results, the simple fact is: The practice of homeopathy RCT results are no better or worse than those of orthodox medicine. Homeopaths have been at the mercy of the (almost obsessed) proponents of the RCT method, who continually and loudly state that homeopathic remedies are no better than placebo.

At the beginning of 2015, results of RCTs of homeopathy showed:

- 41% had a balance of positive evidence,
- 5% had a balance of negative evidence, and
- 54% no conclusions could be drawn either way.[76]

At the beginning of 2015, results of RCTs of orthodox medicine showed:

- 44% of reviews concluded the treatment method studied was likely to be positive,
- 7% the treatment was likely to be negative, and
- 49% reported the evidence was non-conclusive.[77]

These two types of methodology, when treated in RCTs, measure up fairly equally! At the same time, it is important to point out that homeopathic remedies achieve their results while "doing no harm," without dangerous side effects. They also do not increase viral and bacterial resistance, yet improve immunity and well-being.

The bias that is present against homeopathy rages on. We can vent and argue and show evidence endlessly, but it seems the bias is concreted in. And perhaps it stems from an unwillingness to look outside the conventional box. Here is a quote from authors of an article published more than 15 years ago, in the Journal of Alternative and Complementary Medicine, from December 1999:

"We examined two examples of recent articles on complementary and alternative medicine that appeared in two major medical journals in 1998. One is an editorial on the risks of alternative medicine, published in The New England Journal of Medicine and the other is a study on Therapeutic Touch, published in the Journal of the American Medical Association. We evaluated whether information and opinions presented in this editorial and article are objective or not. We found that these examples reflect, at best, misinformation or misunderstanding of the field, or at worst, disingenuousness. We consider the possibility that this apparent bias may be due to the fact that some of the concepts implicit in alternative medicine are outside the current biomedical framework. Yet, it is only by exploring knowledge outside the boundaries of existing dogmas that real (as opposed to incremental) progress can occur."[78]

All these years later, little has changed. The bias remains.

Neutral Switzerland Says Homeopathy Works

We have come to expect neutrality and lack of bias from Switzerland. I was thrilled, several years ago, when the Swiss government released its long-awaited report on homeopathic medicine. The Swiss government stated, in its 2011 report, that after reviewing countless studies, homeopathic treatment is both efficacious and cost-effective. Furthermore, it goes on to recommends that homeopathic treatment be covered by Switzerland's national health insurance program. This stands as the most comprehensive evaluation of the homeopathic practice of medicine ever produced by a government.[79]

I greatly respect the fact, as well, that even though Switzerland is the home and headquarters of several of the world's largest pharmaceutical companies, this did not sway its findings. The highly comprehensive review confirmed that which we homeopaths see in practice day and day out: homeopathic high-potency remedies do cause balancing or normalizing effects on living organisms, and lead to confirmable changes in cells and/or tissues.

Homeopathy and CFS

Many respected homeopathic practitioners have written regarding their clinical findings regarding CFS. Dr. M. Jenkins wrote, in the British Homeopathic Journal, that the most commonly required remedies for ME (CFS) include

Mercurius Sol, Natrum Carbonicum, Kali Phosphoricum, Zincum, Picricum Acidum, Phosphoric Acidum, and Manganum. He went on to discuss his view that although acknowledging the need to choose constitutional remedies for his CFS patients, he felt the syndrome had an organic base.[80] Dr. N.G Dimitriadis, in "Homeopathic Links," reports many successful cases of CFS treatment, including those that did not fit into a symptom picture of a polycrest remedy.[81] Dr. B. Rao, as well, discussed ME in March 1991 edition of Homeopathic Heritage. He emphasizes the part the psoric miasm plays in this syndrome, and lists the most commonly used remedies, in his opinion. They are Phosphoric Acidum, Sabadilla, Sulphuricum Acidum, Veratrum, and Zincum.

In 1995. a questionnaire was sent out to 320 registered UK homeopathic practitioners, 71 of which were returned with some interesting data. The vast majority of these practitioners (69 of 71) felt they had been helpful to their CFS patients, but few felt their cure was fully established. The questionnaire revealed that the practitioners found that if patients were homeopathically treated within 2 years of onset of illness, prognosis was for a 90% recovery. Most respondents felt that constitutional prescribing was the treatment of choice, but stressed the necessity to address miasmatic indications, and deal with acute conditions in a supportive capacity.

In this questionnaire, the remedies that proved to be the most effective were, in descending order of frequency of mention, Carcinosin (14), Phosphoricum Acidum (11), Tuberculinum (7), Gelsemium (6), Natrum Muriaticum (6), Sulphur (5), Pulsatilla (5), Calcarea Carbonica (5), Phosphorus (5), plus 49 other remedies.

This questionnaire confirmed what other practitioners have long found to be true with regard to CFS. The remarkable consensus from these practitioners is that ME (CFS) is a disease, which almost uniformly affects high achievers, who consistently drive themselves, overwork, and are afraid of failure or weakness. A trigger, such as a stressful trauma, death in the family, severe disappointment, or viral illness, can be the last straw in this stressed, often nutritionally deficient person.[82]

In 2004, Weatherley-Jones, etc al, conducted another study into the homeopathic treatment of CFS. It involved 103 patients who received monthly consultations with a homeopathic practitioner, over a six-month period. The results: patients in the homeopathic medicine group showed significantly more improvement in general fatigue. The authors stated, "More people in the homeopathic medicine group showed clinical improvement on all primary outcomes."[83]

Another interesting piece of research is the yearlong study reported in the *International Journal of Alternative and Complementary Medicine* (February through April 1996). This trial was coordinated by Robert Awdry, a member of the

Society of Homeopaths in London. Conducted by the London Homeopathic clinic under the auspices of the London College of Classical Homeopathy, it was overseen by respected homeopathic physicians, academics, and researchers. A randomized, double-blind trial involving 64 patients tested the effectiveness of single selected homeopathic remedies.

The results of the study showed that 33% of those patients taking homeopathic remedies experienced greater improvement than those taking placebos. The response to the remedies was very wide; some patients did not respond at all while others made an almost total recovery. From the response charts of the patients, 20% "recovered," 11% were "largely unchanged," 6% were "slightly better," 4% were "greatly improved," and 30% were "improved." The relapsing nature of this syndrome was noted, even in those who experienced improvement. The younger the patient, the greater was the likelihood of recovery. The shorter the duration of ill health, the greater was the chance of favorable outcome.

In analyzing these results, many thoughts come to mind. Mr. Awdry puts forth the possibility, in his discussion of the study published in the Journal of Alternative and Complementary Medicine, that the "most accurate similimum remedies have not yet been identified."[84] It is also highly possible that life style changes must be made in order to truly effect a cure, especially with regard to the "driven, A-type nature" of most CFS patients. Diet must certainly be investigated, especially with regard to the allergic and Candida-inducing components.

Also, it must be stated that these trials fully tested the abilities of the prescribing homeopathic practitioners, as well as the concept of classical homeopathy itself. It would be very interesting to see studies performed with complex homeopathy as a comparison treatment modality. In my experience, a mixture of the two modalities, plus general health/diet improvements, would effect the greatest improvement in patients.

*The most up-to-date and complete resource for the research into homeopathy is Dana Ullman's ebook entitled, "Evidence Based Homeopathic Family Medicine, available on his website, **www.Homeopathic.com.**

NUTRITIONAL AND HERBAL SUPPORT

Nutrition and Diet

Although a complex area of study in itself, attention to nutritional status is a vital component of any treatment of CFS. One simply cannot discuss the homeopathic treatment of CFS without addressing the diet, and the possible nutritional deficiencies that may be present.

As we look more and more at the advantages of building up the immune system, and practicing preventative medicine, it is becoming apparent that ill health is more to do with the terrain of the body, than to the pathogen. Optimum nutritional status is vital for the health of the physical terrain. If the body has all the nutrients it requires for enzyme function, immune function, etc., and is operating from a correct alkaline/acid balance, it can maintain its own health, fending off attacks from invading microbes. When this terrain is out of balance, it becomes ripe for the many pathogens in our environment to take hold in the body.

With regard to diet, it is essential that CFS patients avoid their known allergens, limit sugar and refined carbohydrates, and eat good quality protein, such as fish and chicken, as a high proportion of CFS sufferers suffer from amino acid deficiency. It is wise that they avoid dairy products, as they are so commonly found to be the cause of allergic reactions.

Dairy products also have an inflammatory response in the body, as they trigger the inflammatory arachadonic prostaglandin pathway. Red meat is another substance that triggers this inflammatory pathway, and should be kept to a minimum. Patients instead should be encouraged to eat more vegetables, salads, low sugar fruits like berries, citrus fruit, plums, etc, and limit refined carbohydrates. This will tend to create the correct alkaline content in the body's terrain, and also discourage the growth of Candida.

All CFS patients should avoid stimulants such as caffeine, and reduce alcohol intake, as it lowers immune activity in the body. The defense system of the chronic fatigue patient is exhausted, and his or her immune system is overactive, fighting a known or unknown assailant. To regain health, it is essential that the patient's environment be as stress-free and toxin-free as possible.

Intestinal treatment must be included in the plan, as dysbiosis is common. Beneficial intestinal flora probiotics such as lactobacillus should be supplemented to discourage Candida overgrowth, and to repopulate the bowel with "good" intestinal bacteria. Digestive enzymes are of great help to some CFS patients, such as betaine hydrochloride, papain, bromelain, pepsin, or digest enzymes derived from aspergillus oryzae. A complete vitamin, mineral, and antioxidant formula should be given, to help support the enzymes of detoxification. This also helps to ensure that the prescribed homeopathic remedies are working in a body that has the necessary nutrients for healing.

Magnesium

Magnesium is the fourth most abundant nutrient in the body, and its deficiency affects many bodily processes. It is an extremely important nutrient with regard to Chronic Fatigue Syndrome, as it is involved in energy production, oxidative phosphorylation, and glycolysis. Magnesium is essential for the synthesis of DNA, RNA, and the glutathione, a powerful antioxidant. [85] It contributes to bone development and plays an essential role in nerve impulse, muscle contraction, and normal heart rhythm.

It is a sad and little-known fact that a majority of Americans are deficient in this vital mineral: a 2005 government study reports a full 68% of Americans do not consume the recommended daily intake of magnesium. [86] [87] CFS sufferers are no exception. A very high percentage of CFS sufferers prove to have intra-cellular magnesium deficiency, and benefit from magnesium injections. [88] [89]

It is important to clarify here that serum (blood) Mg levels are the easiest to measure, but are unreliable, since less than 1% of the total body Mg is in the serum. Most magnesium is intracellular, and this is the level which must be ascertained.

A study reported in the British Journal of Nutrition in
2008 showed that intra-cellular magnesium is significantly
lower in patients with CFS than in controls. This study also
showed that magnesium injections are of considerable benefit
to CFS sufferers, especially to those with muscle aches.[90]
Many doctors are now using injections of Magnesium
Sulfate, and seeing improvement in CFS symptoms.

This injection can unfortunately be somewhat painful and
a small amount of procaine mixed with the Magnesium will
lessen the discomfort. Oral magnesium can also be helpful,
taken either in foods high in magnesium, such as green leafy
vegetables and nuts and seeds, or as capsules of magnesium
threonate or glycinate, the most readily absorbed and utilized
forms of magnesium.

Malic Acid

Another nutrient, best used with magnesium, is malic
acid, (extracted from apples) which in studies has proven to
be effective in reducing pain and inflammation in the muscles
of CFS and Fibromyalgia patients.[91] These two nutrients are
important for the maintenance of energy, as both magnesium
and malic acid are involved in the production of ATP, the
universal energy currency of the body.

Krebs Cycle Nutrients

All of the nutrients involved in the production of energy (the Krebs cycle) may be of benefit to the CFS patient. This includes magnesium, but also carnitine and B12, which have been proven regularly deficient in those with CFS. Coenzyme Q 10 (ubichinone) is also very helpful, as it raises oxygen usage in the body. This can be given both as a nutrient (60mg-100mg per day), and as a homeopathic remedy, in a low-potency such as 6x. Another effective way to stimulate the energy cycle is through the use of combinations of low-potency homeopathics consisting of the constituents of the Krebs cycle itself. Coenzyme Compositum, Ubichinon, and Gallium Heel are such combinations, made by the German company BHI/Heel. For example, particularly useful is Coenzyme Compositum, which consists of 6-8x potencies of Vitamin C, Vitamins B_1, B_2, B_6, B_3, Acidum citricum, Acidum fumaricum, Acidum ketoglutaricum, Acidum malicum, Acidum succinicum, Manganum, Magnesium, Lipoic acid, NAD (Nicotinamid-adenin-dinucleotid) Coenzyme A, and Beta vulgaris rubra.

Vitamin C

Of course, Vitamin C is extremely helpful, as it is in all chronic illness. There are countless studies supporting its use in cases of fatigue, for antiviral and antibacterial properties, for its immune strengthening properties, and for its ability to lower histamine in the allergic patient. It increases the absorption of iron, often a factor in fatigue, especially in menstruating women. Vitamin C also is essential for the production of adrenal hormones, therefore playing a large role in handling stress. Vitamin C is available in high amounts in green and red bell peppers, black currants, kiwi fruit, broccoli, citrus fruits, and strawberries.

It can also be supplemented, ideally in calcium ascorbate form. This is an alkalinized, or buffered form of Vitamin C, which has several advantages over plain ascorbic acid. Calcium ascorbate is better absorbed and utilized, will not contribute to acidity levels in the body, and is easier on the gut. The patient can absorb a much greater level of Vitamin C in alkaline form, before experiencing the gas and diarrhea caused by ascorbic acid.

Trace Minerals (Chromium and Manganese)

The possibility of trace mineral deficiencies must be considered for the CFS patient. Many minerals are often deficient in today's western diet, due to modern chemical farming techniques that fail to replace minerals in the soil, and to the nature of much of our highly processed foods. Iron status must be checked and addressed, as its function in energy is well known and documented.

Two minerals less often remembered by practitioners are manganese and chromium. These minerals are both commonly deficient in the western diet. Manganese is sometimes called "the forgotten mineral," but is involved in no less than twenty enzyme processes in the body, responsible for bone growth, lubrication of joints, sugar balance, and nerve transmission. When deficient in the body, symptoms may include glucose intolerance, reduced brain function, middle ear imbalances, dizziness, and nervous instability such as anxiety. Manganese can be supplemented as a nutrient, and/or as the homeopathic remedy Manganum Aceticum, in our Materia Medica.

Chromium is an essential trace mineral necessary for "glucose tolerance," or the handling of sugar in the blood. It is commonly deficient in today's diet of processed foods, as chromium is a mineral easily lost in processing. Couple this with the fact that so much white sugar, white flour, and quickly digested carbohydrates are being consumed, and chromium, which is essential to the insulin/ blood sugar mechanism, is even more in demand in the body. Studies indicate that this dietary trend has lowered normal human chromium levels in modern Western people compared with 100 years ago, and it is highly possible that this deficiency shows itself in increased heart disease, diabetes, hypoglycemia, and impaired protein metabolism. Chromium, usually 200 mcg daily along with Vanadium, Manganese and Vitamin B3 for sugar metabolism, can be supplemented in CFS patients who have symptoms of hypoglycemia or poor sugar metabolism. Homeopathic Chromium Oxidatum. (low-potency, as in 3x or 6x) can also be used as a tissue salt to more quickly build up the nutrient status of this mineral. With low blood sugar (hypoglycemia) symptoms being so prevalent in CFS patients, many would benefit from supplementation of both the nutrient form of GTF Chromium, and homeopathic Chromium Oxidatum.

Essential Fatty Acids

Another nutrient group that can be considered for supplementation in Chronic Fatigue Syndrome is that of the essential fatty acids, linoleic (Omega 6) and linolenic (Omega 3). These have consistently been shown to decrease inflammation and boost immune function. Good food sources of linoleic oils are flaxseeds, borage oil, oil of evening primrose, and pumpkin seed oils. Fish oils are the prime source of linolenic oils, as well as safflower and sunflower oil. They can also be used in capsule form.

Bioflavinoids

Another group of nutrients that may be considered for the patient suffering from Chronic Fatigue Syndrome are the bioflavinoids. These are found in high amounts in citrus fruits and vegetables, particularly oranges, cherries, grape skins, blackberries, and grapefruit. They act as powerful anti-inflammatory agents, helping to protect the CFS patient from the fatigue caused by allergic reactions. They tend to lower histamine and leukotriene reactions, both producers of inflammation in the body. A specific example of these bioflavinoids is quercetin, which inhibits the release of histamine mast cells in both the digestive and respiratory tracts.

Amino Acids (Phenylalanine and Tyrosine)

For the depression that is so often a part of the Chronic Fatigue Syndrome, one can consider supplementing DL-Phenylalanine (DLPA) and Tyrosine, two amino acids that can often lessen depression. One must of course remember that it is unwise to use either of these amino acids if the patient is taking MAO inhibitors, such as Nardil (phenylzine sulfate) or Parnate (tranylcypromine sulfate).

NADH

NADH, which stands for "5-nicotinamide adenine dinucleotide (NAD) plus hydrogen (H)," is involved in the cycle of energy production. Therefore, it can help in cases of reduced energy, such as CFS. I suggest it be used in tablet form, 5-10 mg per day.

Ginseng

The practitioner can also suggest the use of Siberian Ginseng, (eleutherococcus senticosus). This is one of a group of adaptogens, substances that produce a non-specific supportive or defensive effect on the body, allowing it to handle greater toxicity or stress than it would normally be able to do. These adaptogens have been extensively researched, especially in Russia with regard to the space program. (See also "dysregulation of the hypothalamus-pituitary-adrenal axis" in the appendix section on Endocrinology and CNS Involvement.)

Siberian Ginseng is very helpful in increasing energy, mental concentration, and performance, and is gentler than the more familiar Panax ginseng, which can be over stimulating. Ginseng, as an adrenal support, can be very helpful in adrenal exhaustion, which may be a part of the entire Chronic Fatigue Syndrome picture.

Handling the Case

It must be said that using supplements other than simple vitamins and minerals required by the body can make it somewhat more difficult for the homeopathic prescriber to judge the improvement of the patient. This is due to the fact that symptom relief may be due to amino acid therapy, to Siberian Ginseng, or to another supplement or therapy other than the homeopathic remedy or remedies. This can also be true of using other complementary therapies, such as ozone, exercise, raw glandular concentrates, relaxation and meditation techniques, breathing techniques, etc.

However, the first goal of the practitioner must be to try to aid the patient's recovery, in any way that does no harm. It is possible to employ other therapies and supplements during the course of homeopathic treatment, as long as one bears these other treatment in mind, and allows for the possibility that improvement may be due to one of these concurrent treatments. And as long as the patient is improving, this is the ultimate goal. Most patients do not care how or from where the improvement comes, but are just grateful when it happens.

It is also possible that strict classical homeopaths wish to retain scientific simplicity of treatment, for the benefit of the practitioner. In this way, he or she stands to learn from the course of prescriptions if homeopathic single remedies are the only treatment being pursued. However, I believe that this scientific study is best done in clinical trials, as the patient must be the prime consideration. Besides, there is adequate learning to be obtained from the cure of any patient, no matter how this improvement was achieved.

SUMMARY

*"The number of rational hypotheses that can explain
any given phenomenon is infinite."*

Robert Pirsig, *Zen and the Art of Motorcycle
Maintenance*

Sometimes it seems that those involved in orthodox
medicine simply do not understand this statement. Endless
research to find a single cause for Chronic Fatigue syndrome
may prove to be a futile waste of time and money. Rather
than argue about the possible causes of CFS, homeopaths,
and others in the alternate community are busy unraveling
cases of CFS, layer by layer, allowing the "doctor within" to
resolve and balance the patient.

*"The terrain is everything
the germ is nothing"*
~ Claude Bernard.

*"Bernard was right; the pathogen is nothing;
the terrain is everything."*
~ Louis Pasteur's deathbed admission

As we look more and more at the advantages of building
up the immune system and practicing preventative medicine,
it is becoming apparent that ill health is more to do with the

terrain of the body, than to the pathogen. In other words, if the body is balanced, in nutritional content, acid/alkaline balance, psychological and emotional health, etc., it can maintain its own health, fending off attacks from invading microbes. It is only when this terrain is out of balance and toxic that the pathogens that are a normal part of our environment stand a chance of taking hold in the body. After an entire career spent researching single pathogens, Louis Pasteur, said, on his deathbed, "The pathogen is nothing – the terrain is everything."

Practitioners must use all means at their disposal to help the patient achieve this balance. It may involve tackling CFS from various angles and with all the tools available.

> *"Obviously, the first thing you have to do is to see that it's real. That's not even a question for me anymore. Once you see that it's real, it's a matter of having the right technology and a multidisciplinary approach."* ~ Jose G. Montoya, MD, professor of medicine and infectious diseases at Stanford University Medical Center, and head of Stanford's ME/CFS Initiative.

One must employ the right tool for the job, which may include nosode therapy, classical constitutional work, nutritional and herbal support, gentle exercise, counseling, and even massage and other bodywork. Different modalities work for different patients and it is wise to keep in mind the axiom made famous by Dr. Margarie Blackie, "The patient, not the cure." There may be patients for whom one can never find an absolute cause, but, in my experience, a combination of remedies, either drainage remedies, or single remedies combined, help most patients or clients. Too much exertion, stress, or eating incorrectly can send them into a tailspin, but most of them will regain some control over their lives. With the backup of diet changes, nutrients supplements, herbs, and gentle sustained exercise, I have found that homeopathic remedies, in combination and in single use, are invaluable and essential to the healing effort of the Chronic Fatigue Syndrome patient.

Of all the various healing modalities, homeopathy is the most powerful in the treatment of Chronic Fatigue Syndrome. Correctly chosen homeopathic remedies gently push the patient's system towards optimum balance, leaving the rest to the wisdom of the body and mind to effect the cure.

APPENDIX: INFORMATION & RESOURCES

Theories and Research

Here is a selection of the interesting and possible theories with regard to a cause for Chronic Fatigue Syndrome, backed up by some of the research that has been conducted. For an in-depth study of these areas I recommend Erica Verillo's excellent, *Chronic Fatigue Syndrome: A Treatment Guide, 2nd Edition.*

Viruses (single cause theory)

A large amount of research has been conducted into the potential viral connection with CFS. No less than nine different RNA and DNA viruses have been associated, but the theory that single virus is the culprit has not been proven, although the herpes virus family, enteroviruses, stealth viruses, and retroviruses have all been investigated.[92]

It seems that in many CFS patients, there are elevated titers of Herpes simplex virus 6 (HHV-6), Epstein Barr (EBV), and Coxsackie B,[93] but this picture has been confused by the fact that virus particles are often found in healthy patients, as well. For example, 90% of adults in developed countries have been exposed to EBV by the age of 30.[94]

Perhaps it will be found true that viruses such as Coxsackie or EBV implant themselves in muscles, becoming a "trigger" for Chronic Fatigue Syndrome at some future point of stress.[95] Research into retroviruses, up until now, has not proven they play a substantial role in the pathogenesis of CFS. [96 97 98 99]

Some researchers are looking into a theory of a "hit and run" type of viral infection which leaves the immune system in a continued state of activation after the virus has been eliminated. They have detected an up-regulation of the 2-5-A synthetase RNAse antiviral pathway in patients with Chronic Fatigue Syndrome, and this may support this new theory.[100]

The hope that a single, sole cause of Chronic Fatigue Syndrome will be isolated waxes and wanes. Ten years ago it had been almost completely abandoned, but recently the most attention has been focused on Herpesvirus-6. [101]

If CFS is preceded by infections, there can be long-lasting effects. Dr. Martin L. Pall, Professor of Biochemistry at Washington State University has published a theory regarding CFS and raised levels of nitric oxide and peroxynitrite in response to an infection. He has observed that infections often precede and cause CFS, and these infections create an increased level of inflammatory substances known as cytokines, that produce nitric oxide. This Nitric oxide goes on to produce the potent oxidant peroxynitrite. Peroxynitrite, once created, seems to produce more peroxynitrite, continuing the elevated levels, and therefore the inflammatory symptoms of the patient., in a sort of vicious cycle. According to Dr. Pall, this cycle maintains chronicity of the inflammatory conditions of CFS. [102] [103]

Research in other areas is still in progress, aimed at understanding and finding treatments for this devastating syndrome. The results of the work have been promising, if frustrating. Epidemiological studies show that although there are raised percentages of CFS sufferers with altered immune markers, there is no consistent or constant single marker to diagnose the disorder. In other words, there is still no definite way to diagnose this problem. The CDC in Atlanta is very reticent in the information it makes available, "No diagnostic test exists for CFS. Serologic assays for agents that cause latent or persistent infections have no value in the diagnosis of CFS," and "no characteristic pattern of serum cytokines has been established... The usefulness of activation markers in diagnosing CFS remains to be established."[104]

There have been abnormal changes in some Chronic Fatigue Syndrome patients, sometimes even a rather high percentage, but never in all. For example, there have been abnormal CD4 and CD8 numbers and ratios, abnormal macrophage, B cell, and neutrophil functions, abnormalities in the complement cascade as demonstrated by C3, C4, and Ch50, and IgG subclass deficiencies.[105]

But although studies have found altered immune system markers, the CDC expresses that there is not enough corroboration with other studies to be able to define this condition with a specific test or assay. There is not yet a definitive marker to confirm the diagnosis of CFS/M.E.

Vagus Nerve Infection Hypothesis (VNIH)

In June of 2013, an exciting new hypothesis was published in *Medical Hypotheses* by Michael VanElzakker, a Tufts neuroscientist: CFS may be the result of a pathological infection of the vagus nerve. Vagus Nerve Infection Hypothesis (VNIH) theorizes that an immune response is triggered by a nerve-loving virus or viruses. [106] This produces the cluster of symptoms, including profound fatigue, from which CFS patients suffer.

As well as holding the distinction of being the largest nerve in the body, with roots into almost all human organs, the vagus nerve also connects the immune system to the brain. If the vagus nerve detects pro-inflammatory processes in an organ, such as stomach, lungs, esophagus, etc, it sends signals to the brain to initiate "sickness behavior," such as fever, muscle aches, fatigue, depression, that throbbing flu-like feeling. All the symptoms of Chronic Fatigue Syndrome.

Whether there is found to be a pathogen involved or not, it is true that the increased levels of immune response (i.e.

cytokines such as interleukons, interferons, and tumor necrosis factor) so often found in CFS patients could be the mechanism responsible for the symptoms of Chronic Fatigue Syndrome.[107] [108] These raised levels of cytokines, such as Interleukins I and II, and interferon, boost the immune response, as they are the chemicals that do battle against foreign invaders. And they make us feel pretty dreadful when we have the flu or CFS: they cause fever, malaise, that sense of throbbing, and body aches.

VanElzakker suggests that when the vagus nerve itself is infected with a virus or bacteria, an exaggerated version of sickness behavior can result. The instructions from the brain include telling the body to stop moving, to slow down, to stop eating, or thinking, or exerting.

One of the viruses strongly connected to the nervous system is the herpes virus family. For example, it is one of the herpes viruses, Varicella-Zoster that causes shingles, by infecting the trigeminal nerve. Is it possible, then, as VanElzakker proposes, that a herpes virus infection of the vagus nerve could cause ME/CFS?

Most humans have carried one or more of the herpes viruses such as Epstein Barr (HHV-4), Cytomegalovirus (HHV-5), or HHV6, and these have been thought associated with CFS for many years. The viruses tend to remain in latent form in the body, deep in the nervous system, until there is some as yet undetermined stressor or biological event that reactivates them.

Although VanElzakker proposes that many possible viruses or bacteria could trigger CFS, he is leaning towards the culprit being HHV-6.

However, one of the problems with diagnosing a potential herpes virus infection of the vagus nerve is that they do not test in the blood, and you can't biopsy the vagus nerve in a living person! Hopefully, more research will soon uncover the ways to diagnose this, but in the meantime, VanElzakker is proposing glial cell inhibitors as a standard treatment for CFS, assuming there is a vagus nerve infection. The microglia are cells that surround and protect the neurons in spinal cords and in the brain. When these cells are activated, they begin to release inflammatory and neurotoxic substances that cause sickness behavior symptoms such as mental fogginess, aching, and fatigue.[109]

Drugs which inhibit this response could stop the over-reaction of the immune activation, while practitioners could incorporate anti-virals to attack the viral pathogens. It will be very interesting to see the path and results of further research in this area. Again, this does not address the cause of the CFS, but suffering patients will take what they can get, believe me.

Autoimmunity

Another theory being investigated relates to the autoimmune aspect of Chronic Fatigue Syndrome. A high proportion of CFS sufferers have symptoms of autoimmune activity. Studies looking at blood markers of CFS patients, showed that 52% - 63% of CFS sufferers tested positively for antinuclear antibodies of the IgG isotope [110] and this high frequency of auto-antibodies to insoluble cellular antigens, points to a possible auto-immune component in CFS.[111]

(See also immune system-gut connection in the appendix section called Gut Factor).

Also, if indeed it is finally proven that there is a decrease in T-suppressor cells in CFS sufferers, this could also explain the tendency to autoimmunity, as the level of T-suppressor cells plays an important role in the immune system's self-tolerance.[112] Furthermore, due to uncontrolled toxin damage, the immune system may have to face large amounts of endogenous proteins, which it must eliminate. Tolerance can then break down if the system becomes overwhelmed.

There are several other syndromes that bear some resemblance to Chronic Fatigue Syndrome in symptom complexity, and are also known to affect mostly women in the childbearing years. These are Lupus, Rheumatoid Arthritis, Hashimoto Thyroiditis, and Multiple Sclerosis. These are mainly considered autoimmune disorders, and some researchers speculate that CFS also fits within this category. The increased occurrence of auto-antibodies in the CFS patients (especially antinuclear anti-bodies, or ANA) may suggest that CFS is associated with or the beginning of autoimmune disease." [113] [114]

A New Infectious Agent?

Still looking for a potential single cause of CFS, scientists speculate that an *unknown* agent may be found to cause Chronic Fatigue Syndrome. Researchers wonder whether, in time, a brand new virus may be found to be at the root cause of this illness. However, unless this happens, it seems highly unlikely that a "magic bullet" therapy, an effective single vaccine, will be found to solve this problem. The constellation of symptoms that make up CFS is just too broad.

Mycoplasmas

Another possible single cause of CFS is mycoplasma infection. Recent research confirms infections with mycoplasma is detected in about 50% of patients with CFS and/or Fibromyalgia. (This infection is only seen in about 10% of healthy individuals.)

One interesting area of study has been into mycoplasma infections. Using Polymerase Chain Reaction blood samples from 132 Chronic Fatigue Syndrome Patients were tested for mycoplasma in blood leukocytes. 63% proved positive compared to 9% of controls.[115] This was then compared to Gulf War Illness victims, 50% of whom also test for this mycoplasma infection. The most common organism found in both cases was Mycoplasma fermentans. Another study published in Molecular Cell Probes (Oct. 1998) reported that M. Fermentans was detected in 32% of the Chronic Fatigue Syndrome patients versus 8% in healthy controls.

Dr. Garth Nicolson and his colleagues at the Institute for Molecular Medicine in Huntington Beach, California have been investigating and conducting research into Gulf War Illness, and its close counterparts, Chronic Fatigue Syndrome and Fibromyalgia. These three disorders are very similar in that the complex list of symptoms overlap and are almost identical. All three have chronic fatigue, muscle pain and soreness, gastrointestinal complaints, lymph node swelling and/or pain, joint pain and stiffness, memory loss, etc. [116] Each of these syndromes has a high degree of environmental sensitivity and raised allergic response.

Dr. Nicolson became interested in certain chronic infectious agents that can cause all the above symptoms, especially Molecutes. This is a class of small bacteria (mycoplasmas) that lack cell walls, and are capable of invading several types of human cells and are associated with many human diseases. [117] [118] Examples of diseases caused by such organisms are pneumonia, asthma, rheumatoid arthritis, immunosuppressive disease such as Aids, and genitourinary infections. Using forensic Polymerase Chain Reaction (PCR), blood samples from 132 Chronic Fatigue Syndrome Patients were tested for mycoplasma in blood leukocytes. 63% proved positive compared to 9% of controls.[119] This is being compared to Gulf War Illness victims, 50% of whom also test for this mycoplasma infection. The most commonly occurring mycoplasma he found was Mycoplasma Fermentans, occurring in 50% of the samples. These mycoplasma are intracellular and have a piece of retroviral nucleic acid (similar to HIV-1 Virus) integrated into its DNA genome. According to the work of Dr. Nicolson, these patients responded to 6-week cycles of particular antibiotics: doxycycline, minocycline, ciprofloxacin, azithromycin, and clarithromycin, whereas 6 weeks of doxycycline alone would lead to recovery plus eventual relapse.[120] [121] These mycoplasma infections are not detected by routine laboratory tests, but require tests that involve gene tracking, and forensic PCR. [122]

Hypotension

Scientists and doctors are presenting, researching, and discussing myriad other theories and possible causes of Chronic Fatigue Syndrome. One area is with regard to blood pressure. A high proportion of CFS patients are found to have neurally mediated hypotension, which is a defect in the way the body controls blood pressure. Abnormal upright tilt tests

have shown a lowered blood pressure in many CFS patients,
and an inability to correct blood pressure as well as controls.
16 of 20 members of a Johns Hopkins University study
responded with improved symptoms to treatment with
electrolyte regulating agents and beta-blockers to slow heart
rate.[123] However, this was a small study, and the authors
called for further work to be conducted in this area to
determine whether the hypotension is a cause, or a result, of
the mechanisms of CFS. It is unlikely that hypotension could
turn out to be a *cause* of CFS, but may somehow be a result
of the cascade of toxicity and imbalance in the patient's
system.

Psychological Factors

Another theory still bandied about, although fortunately
less frequently, is that Chronic Fatigue Syndrome is somehow
primarily a psychological problem. Of course, this makes
CFS sufferers see red! Surveys in the 90s revealed that a high
proportion of healthcare practitioners believed CFS to be
primarily a psychological disorder. Although this is changing,
it has been a sad situation for the suffering CFS victim, if not
taken seriously at her doctor's office. Led to feel that this was
in some way her fault.

Studies have shown that CFS patients are primarily A-
type personalities, hard-working perfectionists, and are unlike
the picture of hypochondria or psychosomatic-induced illness

that one sometimes sees in practice. They tend to describe themselves as "action-prone individuals." [124] These people are truly motivated to get better, and rarely have an incentive to remain ill. This makes the theory that CFS is somehow a psychiatric disease even more difficult to swallow. Studies at Mount Sinai Hospital, in New York, by Susan Levine, MD, have shown that CFS patients make more adrenaline, leading to anxiety and panic disorders, as a result of their illness. The important phrase here is "as a result of their illness." But, unlike those diagnosed with primary panic disorder, giving sedatives to CFS patients will only make them feel worse.[125]

Furthermore, the depression that seems to be so common in CFS sufferers is also apt to be a *result* of the illness, rather than an instigating or primary factor of the syndrome. A study of 48 CFS victims, by Lloyd and Wakefield, concluded that the reported depression in CFS patients was a consequence of their illness, not an originating factor.[126] It is also important to realize that recurrent sore throats, fever, and swollen glands, the common symptoms of CFS patients, are not symptoms typically found in those suffering with clinical depression.

Also, a recent study has shown that there may now be a possible marker for CFS that will differentiate CFS and fibromyalgia from depression. The results of this 2002 study showed that beta-endorphin concentrations were significantly *lower* in patients with Chronic Fatigue Syndrome or fibromyalgia syndrome than in normal subjects and depressed patients, while they were significantly *higher* in depressed patients than in controls. The researchers concluded that, "Evaluation of ... cell beta-endorphin concentrations could represent a diagnostic tool for Chronic Fatigue Syndrome and fibromyalgia and help with differential diagnosis of these syndromes versus depression." [127]

However, one cannot eliminate the psychological problem entirely. Great stress just prior to the onset of the illness is very often reported by CFS patients, and many also report a death in the family occurring before their illness. This may indicate that somehow unresolved or suppressed grief may play a part, certainly on the suppression of the patient's immune system. This must be taken into account when prescribing. For example, when considering a homeopathic remedy, it may be appropriate to choose Ignatia during treatment if the practitioner believes that the grief is unresolved, or is a part of the overall picture. An emotional blockage can certainly hamper or even prohibit treatment, and must be reviewed in the larger picture of the case.

Stress Factor

Let's look a little deeper at this stress relation. A surprisingly large proportion of CFS victims report a high level of continuing stress previous to the onset of their illness. Jay S. Goldstein, M.D., believes that the disease is somehow related to the limbic function of the brain, which would explain this frequency of prior stress. [128] The limbic system is an interconnected group of brain structures within the forebrain, and includes parts of the thalamus, hypothalamus, temporal lobe, and frontal lobe cortex. It is associated with emotional behavior and learning, and with nervous system function. This includes heart rate response, sweating, and emotional reactions such as laughing, blushing, and crying. Damage to the temporal lobe and underlying hippocampus can result in memory, learning, and language problems.

In Dr. Goldstein's view, if the limbic system is somehow involved, this could account for the high frequency of reported severe stress in the lives of CFS sufferers, prior to the onset of the illness. Also, perhaps involvement of the limbic system might explain why CFS seems to affect many more unrelated areas of the body than a virus alone could explain.

Perhaps the limbic system involvement could be explained by another observed difference between CFS sufferers and normal healthy people. A great number of CFS patients (78% in one study[129]) show actual structural changes in the brain. NMR tomography detected, in these patients, areas of high signal intensity in the subcorticol regions, with corresponding demyelinization that resembles the lesions seen in the brain of someone suffering from Multiple Sclerosis. Brain magnetic resonance imaging (MRI) data also suggest that there may be an organic abnormality associated with CFS that differentiates these patients from healthy controls.[130]

Another study, using SPECT (single-photon emission computed tomography), found brain abnormalities in 81% of CFS patients.[131] [132] Also, brain perfusion tests indicate hypo perfusion in some brain areas, especially the hypothalamus and brain stem. This differed from the types of changes that have been observed in people with clinical depression.[133]

CFS patients also report a higher level of daily stress than do healthy controls. This leads one to wonder whether they either handle stress less well or somehow perceive stress differently. Researchers in Belgium, concluded that Chronic Fatigue Syndrome and Fibromyalgia patients show a raised frequency of hassles, higher emotional impact and higher fatigue, pain, depression and anxiety levels from daily stress.[134]

Endocrinology and CNS Involvement

Cortisol, and serotonin: A number of the abnormalities found in Chronic Fatigue Syndrome patients may be explained by a dysregulation of the hypothalamus-pituitary-adrenal axis (HPA), a central nervous system disorder. When HPA is functioning correctly, the body remains stable even under physical and psychological stress because of the actions of hormones such as adrenaline and cortisol.

One of the most interesting findings with regard to CFS is to do with cortisol levels in these patients.[135] Studies have

shown that there is a lowered level of cortisol in CFS
sufferers, or mild hypocortisolism.[136] It is unclear at this point
whether it is a primary feature or is one that is secondary to
other factors, but it is highly probable now that
hypocortisolism is contributing to the symptoms of Chronic
Fatigue Syndrome.[137] [138] [139] This may mean there is a
diminished HPA activity leading to this lowered activity of
the adrenal gland.

One of the most informative studies in this area was
conducted in 2001 by the Department of Psychological
Medicine, Institute of Psychiatry and Guy's, King's and St
Thomas' School of Medicine in London.[140] It was set up to
test whether there is a reduced activity of the hypothalamic-
pituitary-adrenal axis in Chronic Fatigue Syndrome and
whether the augmentation of low dose hydrocortisone therapy
could improve the core symptoms of these patients. 37
medication-free CFS patients (versus healthy controls) had a
pituitary challenge test (human CRH) and a hypothalamic
challenge test [either the insulin stress test (n = 16) or D-
fenfluramine (n = 21). The researchers then measured levels
of ACTH and cortisol responses to human CRH, the insulin
stress test, D-fenfluramine, and urinary free cortisol in versus
controls. Their findings showed that urinary free cortisol
levels were lower in the Chronic Fatigue Syndrome group
compared with the healthy group, but that ACTH responses to
pituitary and hypothalamic challenges are intact in Chronic
Fatigue Syndrome. Their research did not confirm previous
findings of reduced central responses in hypothalamic-

pituitary-adrenal axis function or the hypothesis of abnormal CRH secretion in Chronic Fatigue Syndrome.

Along with hypocortisolism and dysregulation of the hypothalamus-pituitary-adrenal axis, studies have shown CFS patients also have abnormal levels of certain neurotransmitters, such as serotonin deficiency.[141] [142] [143] [144] Ongoing research in the area of neuroendocrinology points to a dysregulation of serotonin pathways. This axis can be affected by higher level of cytokines when they cross the blood/brain barrier, acting as neurotransmitters, which can cause mood swings and can influence perceptive ability.[145]

Another finding, some years ago but still relevant, is with regard to homocystine levels. CFS patients have increased concentrations of homocystine in spinal fluid, plus correlating decreased amounts of the vitamin B12.[146] Various other anomalies have been seen, such as abnormal suppression of arginine, abnormal water metabolism (vasopressin secretion), and low growth hormone in these patients. This may explain the fact that there do seem to be problems in blood sugar (hypoglycemia) in a large proportion of patients with CFS. At present, however, there seems to be little consensus among the orthodox establishment on how to use this information regarding these changes seen in the metabolisms of CFS sufferers.

CFS sufferers can often display unusual pupil responses, again signifying serotonin deficiency or mishandling in the brain. They are often sensitive to light, but opticians find no abnormality in routine eye exams. Dr. John Barbur, of City University, London, and Dr. Ian James, Head of Clinical Research at the Royal Free School of Medicine, also in London, are currently researching this area.

Mitochondrial Dysfunction

Work is also going on in the area of metabolic abnormalities. In this area, several changes in mitochondrial function have been demonstrated in those patients with Chronic Fatigue Syndrome. The mitochondria are the vital "power stations" within the cell, which convert fuel into energy. There are several nutrients that act as coenzymes to ensure this process, such as CoQ10 (ubichinone), B vitamins, magnesium, and carnitine. Although no markers have yet been recognized for CFS, these patients seem to have a deficiency of acylcarnitine, from the amino acid carnitine.[147] This is a substance that modulates coenzyme A, and thereby plays an essential role in energy production in the Krebs cycle, which is the energy producing mechanism of the body. This tends to lead to deficiencies in oxidative metabolism with reduced ATP (adenosine triphosphate) concentrations in the cells, which has also been observed in a high percentage of CFS patients.[148]

A 1995 study found that higher carnitine levels even correlate with better functioning, in the CFS patient,[149] and a study from 1997 confirmed the effectiveness of treating CFS patients with oral carnitine.[150] It is possible that infection, whether viral or fungal, in the muscle, may cause a level of damage of mitochondria function within the cell. This leads to the weakness of muscles, the exacerbation from exercise and the lactic acid it produces.

Also contributing to low ATP concentrations could be the lowered levels of magnesium found in so many CFS patients. A high percentage of CFS sufferers prove to have intra-cellular magnesium deficiency, and benefit from magnesium injections.[151] [152] Many doctors are using injections of Magnesium Sulfate, and seeing improvement in CFS symptoms. This injection can unfortunately be somewhat painful and a small amount of procaine mixed with the Magnesium will lessen the discomfort.

Environmental Toxins

These include mercury and other heavy metal toxicity, pesticide poisoning, and atmospheric pollutants. Many types of toxins can damage the immune system, such as aluminum, mercury, cadmium, nickel, arsenic, dioxin, a wide range of herbicides, pesticides, insecticides and industrial pollutants.

Let us first look at heavy metal toxicity. The poisonous metals, lead, mercury, cadmium, and aluminum have no biological role in the body, and interfere with normal metabolic functions, mainly by interfering with enzyme processes. Nickel, arsenic and copper are also very toxic at high levels. Many researchers and experts in Chronic Fatigue Syndrome consider toxic metal poisoning to be a possible contributing factor in CFS.

There are many potential sources. Dentistry, environmental pollution, lead paints, lead in petrol, aluminum in household products and cookware, and contaminated seafood can all be sources of contamination. Other sources are poultry or livestock additives, wood preservatives, and wallpaper dyes. Many symptoms of heavy metal toxicity are similar to those of CFS, such as unexplained severe fatigue, depression, constipation, diarrhea, difficulty with memory, skin irritations, disturbed sleep, headaches after eating, and abdominal bloating.[153] This prevalence of toxic metals must be held uppermost in the practitioner's mind, and investigated during the course of working with the CFS patient, to ensure that this toxicity is not present.

Mercury is a prevalent problem due to the thousands of silver/mercury fillings placed by dentists every day around the world. Mercury is covered in depth earlier in this book in the section entitled "Mercury Fillings."

Lead toxicity, although less common now that it has been removed from the majority of gasoline supplies around the world, is still pervasive. Although blood levels of lead have declined since the late 1970s, due to phased-out leaded gasoline and lead paint, the National Academy of Sciences states that 600,000 tons of lead is dumped into the atmosphere each year.[154] It is still present in dust and dirt, in drinking water, due to lead pipes in the plumbing of older houses, in canned fruits and juices, in organ meats such as liver, and is available from glazed pottery we may use. It is found in older house paint, bone meal, in pencils, and is even found in milk taken from cows that have grazed on lead contaminated pastures. It will be many years before lead has disappeared from our environment.

Unfortunately, the symptoms of lead toxicity can be very similar to the symptoms of Chronic Fatigue Syndrome; chronic fatigue, headache, depression, insomnia, nervousness, irritability, dizziness, confusion and disorientation, muscle weakness and wasting, aching muscles, bones and joints, abdominal pain and constipation, anemia, and adrenal gland impairment, leading to weakness. And to make matters worse, it is rare that doctors consider the possibility of lead toxicity. Therefore, it is hard to speculate how many patients diagnosed with CFS, who continue to suffer without further intervention, may indeed be lead toxic. This must certainly be eliminated before any diagnosis of CFS can be made. Blood levels are not necessarily an adequate test for lead, as it can be stored in the bones, and therefore is not revealed in blood samples. It is better, therefore, to test for all toxic minerals (heavy metals) with hair mineral analysis, Voll testing, and/or diagnostic chelation. This method uses intravenous EDTA to pull minerals from the body, which can then be accurately tested in the urine as they are eliminated. Chelation therapy itself is a good way to reduce the lead load in the body (and the other toxic heavy metals), but minerals must be supplemented while this is occurring, to prevent mineral deficiency.

Chemical pollutants are other, usually man-made, environmental toxins, which poison the human system. Examples are gases that contaminate the atmosphere, such as carbon monoxide, from auto exhaust, cigarette smoke, and smog. The toxicity symptoms of carbon monoxide are anemia, angina, asthma, bronchitis and other respiratory disorders, headaches, and memory loss. Nitrogen dioxide, also occurring in smog, causes respiratory disorders and cancer. Ozone is also in smog, and can also cause respiratory problems such as emphysema, and cancer. Ozone is a necessary and desirable substance in our atmospheric layer, which only becomes a dangerous substance when it adheres to the toxins that create smog.

Another chemical pollutant in the form of atmospheric gas is the group of polynuclear aromatic hydrocarbons, in smoke from wood, coal, oil, tobacco, and commercial incense. Evidence shows these are carcinogenic substances. Tobacco smoke occurs from the use of cigars, cigarettes, pipes, and leads to lung problems including cancer, and immune disorders. Tobacco smoke also carries hexavalent chromium, which can cause cancer and gastrointestinal problems.

Finally there are the industrial chemicals, such as DDT, PCPs, dioxin, etc, which are in air, water, soil, food, and plant and animal tissues. These can lead to vitamin depletions. Obviously then they can indirectly lead to many forms of illness, including Chronic Fatigue Syndrome.

CFS, Multiple Chemical Sensitivity, & Fibromyalgia

Some researchers are speculating that CFS and Multiple Chemical Sensitivity (MSC) and Fibromyalgia (FM) are the same illness. First, let us look at Multiple Chemical Sensitivity. It has also been called "Environmental Illness," and "Universal Reactor Syndrome." Its symptoms are very like those of CFS: fatigue, flu-like symptoms, mental confusion, and all kinds of skin, urinary, joint, and muscle problems. Some clinicians feel that MCS is a type of Chronic Fatigue Syndrome. It can be provoked by chemical exposure, from such chemicals as formaldehyde, lacquers, plastics, etc. While it is true that many Chronic Fatigue Syndrome patients suffer from allergic reactions to chemicals, not all do, meaning that it is unlikely that CFS and MCS are one and the same. It is more apt to be that some patients with CFS also develop Multiple Chemical Sensitivity, perhaps due to an extreme autoimmune reaction, induced in some way by the as yet unknown mechanisms of CFS.

Fibromyalgia, or Fibromyalgia Syndrome (FMS), also known as fibrositis, was first described in the nineteenth century, and is similar in symptoms to Chronic Fatigue Syndrome. Patients diagnosed with this painful problem experience tender points, called trigger points, along various muscles, soft tissue pain, fatigue, and even similar sleep disturbances and immune system abnormalities to CFS. Both syndromes have a strong chronicity factor, and seem primarily to affect young female adults who have relatively normal laboratory test results. One of the primary differences between the two syndromes is that FMS is alleviated and ameliorated by exercise and stretching, whereas those suffering with CFS will be exacerbated by exercise, even thrown into complete relapse, which can last for days. Also, for the sake of differentiation, in CFS, the fatigue element is usually the greatest, whereas in FMS, the muscular pains are greatest. One final differentiating factor was isolated in a recent, 1997 study in Boston, Massachusetts. Patients with Fibromyalgia were discovered to have reduced levels of somatomedin C (insulin –like growth factor), whereas those with CFS were found to have elevated levels.[155] This anomaly has not yet been satisfactorily explained. However, since somatomedin is secreted in response to exercise (as well as to stress or severe hypoglycemia) it is possible that this may help explain the exercise-induced exacerbation in CFS, and the improvement from exercise for FM patients.

A study by Buchwald and Farrity compared patients with CFS, Multiple Chemical Sensitivity (MSC) and Fibromyalgia

(FM). Their data showed that between 46% to 67% of the CFS and FM patients reported that their symptoms worsened when they were exposed to pollution/exhaust fumes/cigarette smoke/gas/paint, etc.[156] So, nearly half or more of people with Chronic Fatigue Syndrome or Fibromyalgia experience symptoms in reaction to exposure to various chemicals. Furthermore, in this study, 70% of the patients with a FMS diagnosis, and 30% of those with multiple chemical sensitivities met all the criteria for CFS as required by the CDC. The conclusion of the researchers was, "The demographic and clinical factors do not clearly distinguish patients with CFS, FMS, and MCS. Symptoms typical of each disorder are prevalent in the other two conditions."[157] It is indeed likely that although a large proportion of CFS sufferers report symptoms of MCS and FM, these chemicals are not the sole cause of the CFS. Instead there may be an increased allergic response mechanism since the onset of their illness, or a genetic predisposition to this allergic response.

The Gut Factor

Food Allergies

The question raised by these various studies into FMS, CFS and MCS is apparent: are the allergy factors in CFS the cause, or the result of, the illness? It is possible that intestinal malabsorption, or immune system over-reactivity, may bring on the allergic state from which so many CFS patients suffer.

The high prevalence of bowel disturbance in those suffering with CFS was shown in a study[158] conducted at St. Bartholomew's Hospital in London. This found that 63% of the 1,797 CFS patients questioned fulfilled the criteria for irritable bowel syndrome.

The function of the digestive tract contributes in many ways to overall health, in mucus secretion, gastric acid secretion, water and electrolyte secretion, and peristalsis (movement and contraction of the muscles of the bowel) for removal of feces. However, less well known and accepted is the fact that the intestinal tract plays a powerful role in immune function. The immune system of the intestines is extremely extensive, as approximately 40-50% of the body's lymphoid cells line the intestinal tract. The gut mucosal immune system is the first line of defense against the many antigens and pathogens that enter the body via the digestive system.

There is definitely a connection that can be made between allergy and the myalgia (muscle pain) of CFS. That allergic responses cause muscle pains is not a new theory; in the 1920s and 1930s, Dr. A. H. Rowe conducted research that showed that chronic muscular pain had an allergic origin.[159] These pains were associated with weakness, headaches, gastrointestinal symptoms, nausea, mental confusion and drowsiness, irritability, despondency, and widespread body aches. [160]

Consider this possible scenario: a patient experiences continued stress, which lowers the immune system, leaving him vulnerable to, for example, an infection or parasite in the gut. This leads to an increase in gut permeability, a condition in which the gastrointestinal mucosa becomes perforated by tiny holes, permitting absorption of toxins, such as undigested proteins, that would otherwise remain in the lumen. The body's immune defenses attack these undigested toxins as invaders, causing a systemic allergic reaction. Plus, the toxins and antibodies may reach the liver by way of the portal vein and add an additional burden on the detoxification system. The overactive immune reaction then produces cytokines (interferon and interleukins) which cause the symptoms of muscle pain. The cytokines can also create brain dysfunction, which can lead to altered limbic function, altered sleep patterns and temperature control, changes in mood, severe fatigue, lowered pain tolerance and disrupted digestive function. These immune markers, interferon and interleukins, are raised in viral and bacterial reactions, and, when raised, they cause the patient to feel like he or she continually has the flu. This is just one possible path that can lead to the symptoms, and diagnosis, of CFS.

Accepting the degree of food intolerance seen in CFS patients, it begs the question: is it the cause of CFS? Or are food intolerances a side symptom of CFS? Some researchers are speculating that CFS is an autoimmune disease which centers in the gut.

Research into gut involvement in CFS

Let's look for a moment at the probiotics-gut flora connection in CFS. Probiotics have long been a staple addition in alternative and complementary practitioners' protocols, to ease the digestive disturbances from which their CFS patients so often suffer. This was backed up rather nicely in 2009, when a study showed a promising use of probiotics, in this case 24 billion colony-forming units of *Lactobacillus case*. In the randomized study, 39 CFS patients received either the probiotics or a placebo, daily, for two months. At the end of the two months, the CFS sufferers who were taking the probiotics showed a significant decrease in anxiety symptoms, versus the controls.[161]

This anxiety is often connected to a hypersensitivity of the system in CFS patients. It appears this may be caused in part by repeated stress, so often at play in the history of the CFS patient. There is a very interesting finding called "Limbic kindling." This is a condition where either repeated neurological exposure to a stimulus that should not produce problems can lead to hypersensitivity to that same stimulus. So perhaps prolonged and repetitive stress can create hypersensitivity. Add to that the fact that studies show activated nervous systems such as this can lead to gut flora regulation, called dysbiosis.[162] [163] And there is a strong connection already made in the literature that CFS patients often have gut dysbiosis and leaky gut.[164] At the time of writing, there are several interesting studies currently running in the arena of the gut-CFS connection, and results are expected this year. One is from the "Solve ME/CFS Initiative" looking into what effect exercise has on gut flora. Also, Rebecca Hansen's NIH-funded study on microbiome and inflammation is due to be completed this year. It is examining bacterial composition of both the blood and the gut. There is also a study due for publication this year by the Lipkin/Chronic Fatigue Initiative/Microbe Discovery, which is attempting to identify bacteria, viruses, and fungi in stool samples from 100 CFS patients.

So as you can see, there is some promising research underway or imminent for publication.

Multi-Factorial Causes

Although this is changing, slowly, many operating within the world of allopathic medicine and scientific research still seem incapable of grasping a multi-factorial picture with regard to CFS or most other chronic illnesses. They are still influenced by the Newtonian theories of the 17th century, still viewing science as completely explainable in purely mechanical terms. However, it is clear, thanks to the new concepts of relativity and quantum physics, that physical matter and energy are interchangeable and interdependent. The human body simply does not follow a linear pattern of "if A then B." This linear thinking is woefully inadequate in the light of the fact that many chronic illnesses are syndromes, involving several problems, not single-disease entities caused by one lone pathogen. A drug designed to destroy one pathogen may never be a "cure" in something as complicated as Chronic Fatigue Syndrome.

Under this multi-factorial "umbrella" there are many theories being investigated. Sometimes there is more than one microbe involved in the CFS pattern, leading some practitioners and physicians who specialize in treating patients with CFS to label this occurrence as "Mixed Infection Syndrome." Besides viruses such as Epstein Barr,[165] Cytomegalovirus, Herpes Virus 6, Coxsackie (especially "B"), the most commonly found infectious organisms in the CFS patient are yeast (Candida Albicans or Parapsilosis infection) and parasites, most often Giardia Lamblia and Entamoeba histolytic. Dr. Ronald Hoffman, a New York City specialist in chronic fatigue, writes in his book, *Tired all the Time*, "CFS is probably due to a mysterious and highly individual mélange of viruses, yeast, chemical and heavy-metal poisons, and stress." [166] The typical CFS case can be likened to an onion, which presents to the practitioner in layers that need to be peeled away.

Let's take a possible example of CFS. A typical patient may have contracted a parasite, plus have a level of Candida overgrowth, with the metabolic and digestive disturbances brought on by these two problems. Oxidation becomes reduced, and there is an increase in toxicity throughout the system. Throughout this scenario there may be great stress, which can further weaken the immune system. An overloaded lymphatic system then is incapable of protecting itself from a virus, such as Coxsackie B or Cytomegalovirus, which becomes the last straw. And of course it is essential to realize that the last straw is only that, *the last straw*. It is rarely the entire causative factor in something as complex as CFS, and addressing only the "last straw" will not address the whole syndrome. The biological terrain of the body must be addressed, and attention paid to all the possible pathogens or imbalances involved in each case.

Unfortunately, two areas often presenting in Chronic Fatigue Syndrome, parasites and Candida, are not being researched in the orthodox world. Many allopathic physicians, believing these problems to be rarely seen in practice, tend to react with some disdain to the suggestion of the presence of these opportunists.

Rituximab Trials

Rituximab is a cancer medication that targets and eliminates B-cells, cells implicated in autoimmune disease[167] [168] It works by destroying B cells, and is used to treat diseases with overactive, excessive, or in some way dysfunctional B cells. These diseases are leukemias, some types of lymphoma, transplant rejection, and some of the autoimmune disorders, such as rheumatoid arthritis. It must be given in IV form, is extremely expensive, and causes some serious side effects.

However, recent trials have shown symptom relief for a proportion of CFS sufferers with this prescription drug, Rituximab, Two doctors in Norway who specialize in cancer therapies, Dr. Øystein Fluge and Professor Olav Mella, received successful results in their 2011 clinical trial of Rituximab with CFS/ME patients. A full 67% if the study participants recorded moderate to major improvement in their symptoms, as compared to 13% of the controls.[169]

Rituximab works by temporarily wiping out the B-cells of the immune system, which are involved in autoimmune disease. This adds further evidence to the theory that CFS/ME is an autoimmune syndrome. The current 2015 larger study being conducted in Norway will be followed closely, with great anticipation, by patients and doctors alike.[170]

Of course, this kind of targeted treatment comes with various down sides. The drug is extremely expensive, and can cause serious side effects such as headache, stomach pain, chills, fever, nausea, diarrhea, heartburn, flushing, night sweats, weakness, muscle or joint pain, back pain, or dizziness. Plus, the patient taking Rituximab is warned that she may experience a decrease in blood cells (cytopenia) which can cause bleeding problems, and also that there may be a reduction in resistance to other infections.

These side effects are frightening, but more to the point, Rituximab does not address the underlying cause. It eliminates B-cells that are there for a reason. And, it may well cause additional health problems down the line that we are not aware of at this point. Using it for CFS, at this point, seems to be premature.

However, I certainly understand (full well!) that the CFS patient is desperate during this struggle to find anything at all that will help. If this drug relieves symptoms, it is hard to imagine denying it to the suffering patient.

Exercise

One of the criteria for a diagnosis of CFS is that exercise exacerbates. Studies confirm that after moderate exercise, CFS patients show significantly reduced oxygen consumption and altered gene expression.

However, some doctors feel that graded exercise can be beneficial. Dr. Majid Ali, states, in his book, *The Canary and Chronic Fatigue*, "CFS requires holistic, integrated, nontoxic, non-drug, nutritional and environmental therapies. Training in effective methods of self-regulation, and slow, sustained exercise for restoring normal energy patterns is absolutely necessary."[171] Although exertion can bring on relapses of CFS, even in an almost completely recovered patient, gentle slow exercise is vital to the recovery process, due in part to the movement of lymph achieved by gentle exercise. Dr. Ronald Hoffman, a New York specialist in Chronic Fatigue Syndrome, and author of *Tired all the Time*, agrees. He encourages his CFS patients to use what he terms "pulsed exercise," which consists of short cycles of no more than four minutes, walking, cycling, rowing etc., then rest until the pulse returns to normal. He suggests trying to achieve 30 minutes a day of this pulsed exercise, believing that this type of exercise will "reset the autonomic nervous system, taking it out of the cycle of exhaustion and tension and returning it to a healthy cycle of energy and rest."[172]

And studies are beginning to confirm: one study published in the British Medical Journal showed that 35 of 47 CFS patients rated themselves as better one year after supervised, graded, aerobic exercise treatment.[173] This is very difficult for most sufferers of CFS, as they are sometimes too exhausted to walk to the bathroom, let alone exercise. However, if possible, the gentle exercise can be a great help in reestablishing normal Krebs cycle activity of energy production in the body.

That gentle exercise may contribute improvement for CFS sufferers was confirmed again in the well-known (if controversial) PACE study in the UK in 2011.[174] This trial, with 641 CFS patients, showed that graded exercise coupled with cognitive behavior therapy can be helpful.

Of course CFS organizations warn that exercise can exacerbate, often substantially, so this area of treatment must be handled with great care.

RESOURCES

Homeopathic remedies

1) **Ainsworth, (Homeopathic Pharmacy)_**in London. Phone 011 44 71 935 5330. For me, these folks are the kings of homeopathic remedies. They have a large list of nosodes and all single homeopathic remedies in a variety of forms including mother tinctures and 95% alcohol dropper bottles. You can buy them in small, high alcohol bottles from which to make your own remedies to dispense, rather than trying to deal with the expense and time involved in shipping from the UK. http://www.ainsworths.com

2) **Homeopathic.com**. Single remedies, remedy kits, combination remedies, books, audio, learning courses- the works! Great site:

Homeopathy Educational Services
812 Camelia St., Berkeley, CA, 94710

3) Here is a good US homeopathic pharmacy I often frequented when I lived in southern California: **Santa Monica Homeopathic Pharmacy**, 310 395-1131.

4) **Noma,** another company in London (011 44 703 770513) has books, test sets, phenolics, Pascoe and Kern

remedies, acupuncture items, Vega equipment, the "absorber" to wear when testing to help protect you, flower essences, etc. http://www.complementary-medicine.com/

5) I use many **BHI/Heel** products, which are German remedies available here. http://www.heel.com/ These are high quality combination remedies. Sold by Swanson Vitamins and others online: **Swanson.**
http://www.swansonvitamins.com/heel-usa?SourceCode=INTL095&CAPCID=42986469367&cadevice=c&gclid=CjwKEAjwhbCrBRCO7-e7vuXqiT4SJAB2B5u7oxnMEv9pYg7_xwSip9jbqQl8ise9gPSLCJqbeWboiBoC8kjw_wcB&CA_6C15C=5300024600000 83631

6) **Marco Pharma** has great remedies and herbal combinations too, and test kits available. Phone 800 999 3001. Their "Hepatica," which is an herbal drainage remedy for the liver, is terrific, and I highly recommend many of their great products: Thuja, Crataegus, ABC, Viscum (for oral chelation), and Absinthium... plus others! https://marcopharma.com/

7) A terrific source for homeopathic combination remedies is **Deseret Biologicals**, in Utah. They carry phenols as well, and pesticides, in homeopathic form for desensitizing. I can recommend their Metox for mercury detox, plus Neuro 1 and Neuro 2 (these are combination

homeopathic neurotransmitters such as serotonin and dopamine homeopathically), plus many others. http://desbio.com/

8) One of the largest manufacturers of homeopathic remedies is the European company, **Boiron and its subsidiary, Dolisos.** These remedies are widely available at health food stores. http://www.boiron.com/

9) Another good company is **Apex Energetics**, for homeopathic combination remedies and flower remedies.)

10) Miscellaneous: Empty dropper bottles, books, glassware, supplies: **Natural Health Supply**, Jim Klemmer's company in Santa Fe, New Mexico. Phone: (888) 689-1608, or (505) 474-9175. He has a large homeopathic book selection. http://www.apexenergetics.com/

Other Useful Websites

National Institutes of Health:
http://www.nhl.nih.gov/medlineplus

https://vsearch.nlm.nih.gov/vivisimo/cgi-bin/query-meta?query=cfs&v%3Aproject=nlm-main-website

Center for Disease Control and Prevention:
http://www.cdc.gov/cfs

Cort Johnson: http://www.cortjohnson.org

Also from Cort: **Phoenix Rising** http://phoenixrising.me/

Simmaron Research: Scientifically Redefining ME/CFS:
http://simmaronresearch.com/2013/12/one-theory-explain-
vagus-nerve-infection-chronic-fatigue-syndrome/

Homeopathic.com. The most up-to-date and complete
resource for the research into homeopathy is Dana Ullman's
ebook entitled, *"Evidence Based Homeopathic Family
Medicine,* available on his website, ***www.Homeopathic.com.***

CFS Treatment Centers and Clinics

CFS Treatment Guide Website:
http://www.cfstreatmentguide.com/doctors-and-clinics.html

CFS/M.E. Associations:

CFS Treatment Guide Website: National and International CFS/ME Organizations:
http://www.cfstreatmentguide.com/national-and-international-cfsme-organizations.html

Training

British Institute of Homeopathy
http://www.bihint.com/

Occidental Institute

The **Occidental Institute** in Vancouver, B.C., founded by the late Dr. Walter Sturm, has weekend training courses in E.A.V., and sells RM10s (like the Dermatron). They also sell the wonderful "Mora" from Mora 3 to the computerized Mora (goodness knows how much that one is!) Also blank test kits, and books and manuals on E.A.V. I trust regularly to the big black bible; this is the manual of EAV, a big, ringed binder with the points, and remedies to test against them– an education in itself. Phone 250 490 3318. http://www.oirf.com/res-dxtxinfo.html

BIBLIOGRAPHY

Articles or Studies

- Kato K, Sullivan PF, Evengard B, Pedersen NL.
  Premorbid predictors of chronic fatigue. *Arch Gen Psychiatry* 2006 63:1267-72.

- Tucker, Miriam, "Wrong Name, Real Illness." January 8, 2015. *Medscape Rheumatology.* Web
  http://www.medscape.com/viewarticle/837577

- Johnson, Cort, " The CDC's Chronic Fatigue Syndrome Multisite Studies" *Simmaron Research*, Nov 8, 2014. Web.
  http://simmaronresearch.com/2014/11/going-grassroots-dr-unger-cdcs-chronic-fatigue-syndrome-multisite-studies/

- Medline Plus Medical Encyclopaedia. National Institutes of Health; c1997-2009 [cited 2009 February 23]. Chronic Fatigue Syndrome; [about 3 reens]. Available
  from:http://www.nlm.nih.gov/medlineplus/ency/article/001244.htm

- Tuller, David, " Brains of People with Chronic Fatigue Syndrome Offer Clues About Disorder." Nov 24, 2014.

http://well.blogs.nytimes.com/2014/11/24/brains-of-people-with-chronic-fatigue-syndrome-offer-clues-about-disorder/

- Arnold LM, Keck PE, Welge JA. Antidepressant treatment of fibromyalgia. A meta-analysis and review. *Psychosomatics* 2000; 41: 104-113.

- Heim C, Wagner D, Maloney E, et al. Early adverse experience and risk for Chronic Fatigue Syndrome. *Arch Gen Psych* 2006;63: 1258-66.

- Mihaylova I, DeRuyter M, et. al., "Decreased expression of CD69 in Chronic Fatigue Syndrome in relation to inflammatory markers: Evidence for a severe disorder in the early activation of T lymphocytes and natural killer cells." *Neuro Endocrinol Lett.* 2007;28:477-483.

- Prins, JB, van der Meer, JW, et al. "Chronic Fatigue Syndrome." Lancet. 2006 Jan 28;367(9507):346-55. http://www.thelancet.com/journals/lancet/article/PIIS0 140-6736%2806%2968687-X/fulltext?version=printerFriendly

- Whiting P, Bagnall A-M, Sowden AJ, Cornell JE, Mulrow CD, Rameriz G. Interventions for the treatment and management of CFS. A systematic review. JAMA 2001;286:1360-8.

- CDC Program updates ad strategies 2004-2005
  http://www.cdc.gov/cfs/programs/cdc_research/progra
  m_update_2004-2005.html

- Mawle, Nisenbaum, et al, "Seroepidemiology of
  Chronic Fatigue Syndrome: A Case-Control Study, "
  Clinical Infectious Diseases, volume 21, 1997, pgs
  1386-1389

- "Toward a Clearer Diagnosis of Chronic Fatigue
  Syndrome" April 4, 2014 Web
  http://www.sciencedaily.com/news/health_medicine/c
  hronic_fatigue_syndrome/

- Y. Nakatomi, K. Mizuno, et al. "Neuroinflammation
  in Patients with Chronic Fatigue Syndrome/Myalgic
  Encephalomyelitis: An 11C-(R)-PK11195 PET
  Study." *Journal of Nuclear Medicine*, 2014;
  DOI: 10.2967/jnumed.113.131045

- Maquet, D, Demoulin, C., et al. "Chronic Fatigue
  Syndrome: a Systematic Review." *Ann Readapt Med
  Phys.* 2006 Jul;49(6):337-47, 418-27. Epub 2006 Apr
  19.
  http://www.ncbi.nlm.nih.gov/pubmed/16698108

- Afari, N., Buchwald, D. "Chronic Fatigue Syndrome:
  a Review." *Am J Psychiatry.* 2003; Feb;160(2):221-
  36. http://www.ncbi.nlm.nih.gov/pubmed/12562565

- Clague, J., et al. "Intravenous magnesium loading and Chronic Fatigue Syndrome." *Lancet* 1992; 340: 124-125

- Cox, I. "Red Blood Cell Magnesium and Chronic fatigue syndrome" *Lancet* 1991; 337: 757-60

- Dobbins, Natelson, et al, "Physical, Behavioral, and Psychological Risk Factors for Chronic Fatigue Syndrome: A Central Role For Stress?" *Journal of Chronic Fatigue Syndrome,* volume 1, 1995, pgs 43-58

- Mycoplasmas: Sophisticated, Reemerging, and Burdened by their Notoriety," *Emerging Infectious Diseases,* Vol 3, Jan-Mar 1997.

- Gunn, Komaroff, Bell et al, "Inability of Retroviruses to Identify Persons with Chronic Fatigue Syndrome" (49,665 byte .PDF file), *Morbidity and Mortality Weekly Report*, volume 42, 1993, pgs 183-190

- Heneine, Walid and Folks, "Retroviruses and Chronic Fatigue Syndrome," Thomas, from *Chronic Fatigue Syndrome*, S.E. Strauss, editor, Marcel Dekker, Inc., 1994, pages 199-206

- Khan, Heneine, Chapman et al, "Assessment of Retrovirus Sequence and other Possible Risk Factors for the Chronic Fatigue Syndrome in Adults," *Annals of Internal Medicine*, volume 118, pgs 241-245.

- Landay, Alan, et al. "Chronic Fatigue Syndrome:
  Clinical Condition Associated with Immune
  Activation." *The Lancet* 339, no. 8769 (Sept 21,
  1991): pgs 707-711

- Mawle, Nisenbaum, et al, "Immune Responses
  Associated with Chronic Fatigue Syndrome: A Case
  Controlled Study," *Journal of Infectious Diseases*,
  volume 175, 1997, pgs 136-141

- Read, Margaret, "Flavinoids; Naturally Occurring
  Anti-inflammatory Agents," *American Journal of
  Pathology*, August 1995: 147 (2): 235-237

- Puri BK, Counsell SJ, Zaman R, Main J, Collins AG,
  Hajnal JV, Davey NJ Relative increase in choline in
  the occipital cortex in Chronic Fatigue Syndrome.
  Acta Psychiatr Scand 2002 Sep;106(3):224-226

- Reyes, Gary, Dobbins, et al, "Descriptive
  Epidemiology of Chronic Fatigue Syndrome: CDC
  Surveillance in Four Cities" *Morbidity and Mortality
  Weekly Report Surveillance Summaries,* Feb 21, 1997,
  Volume 46 / No. SS-2, pgs 1-13

- Reyes, Dobbins, Mawle, Steele, et al, "Risk Factors
  for Chronic Fatigue Syndrome," *Journal of Chronic*

Fatigue Syndrome, volume 2, pgs 17-33

|

- Smit, Dr. Alta, "Chronic Fatigue Syndrome- A Homotoxological View," *Biologische Medizin*; 1996 August: 159-65

- Steel, Dobbins, Fukuda et al, "The Epidemiology of Chronic Fatigue in San Francisco," *American Journal of Medicine*, 1997

- Theodorou V, Ficramonti J, Bueno, L. Integrative neuroimmunology of the digestive tract. (Ecole Suppaerieure D'Agriculture de Purpan, Toulouse, France) *Vet Res*, 1996, 27: 4-5, 427-42

- Walker, Morton, "Metallic Toxicity as a Cause of the Downhill Syndrome," *Townsend Letter for Doctors*, #160; Nov 1996; pages 116-122

- Van der Hulst, RR, von Meyenfeldt MF, et al. *Journal of Parenteral Nutrition* Nov, 21:6, 310-5

Books

- Banerjee, PN, *Chronic Disease- Its Cause and Cure*, B. Jain Books, India, 1931

- Bellavite P, MD, Signorini A, *The Emerging Science of Homeopathy*, North Atlantic Books, Berkeley California; 2002

- Boericke, William, *Materia Medica with Repertory*, B. Jain Publishers, New Delhi, India, reprint 1990

- Burnett, James Compton, *Best of Burnett*, B. Jain Publishers, New Delhi,1900

- Chaitow, Leon, Vaccination and Immunization: Dangers, Delusions and Alternatives, CW Daniel, Saffron Waldon, Essex, England, 1987

- Chaitow, Leon, *Postviral Fatigue Syndrome*, JM Dent and Sons, London, 1989

- Chaitow, Leon, *Vaccination and Immunization*, The C.W. Daniel Company, Saffron Waldon, England, 1987

- Crook, W. M.D. *Chronic Fatigue and the Yeast Connection. Jackson,* TN: Professional Books, 1992

- Edwards David, MD HMD, and Ibarra, Corazon, MD HMD *An Introduction to Homotoxicolgy* , Menaco Publishing, 1998

- Farrington E.A., *Clinical Materia Medica,* B. Jain Publishers, New Delhi, reprint 1994

- Gittelman, Ann Louise, *Guess What Came To Dinner*, Avery Publishing, Garden City, New York, 1993

- Hoffman, Ronald, *Tired all the Time*, Simon and Simon, N.Y., N.Y., 1993

- Hoffman, Ronald L., MD, Intelligent Medicine; A Guide to Optimizing Health and Preventing Illness for the Baby-Boomer Generation, Fireside, Simon & Schuster Inc., New York, New York 1997

- Huggans, Hal, *It's All in Your Head,* Avery Publishing, Garden City, New York, 1993

- Kroeger, Hanna, *Parasites, The Enemy Within*, 7075 Valmont Drive, Boulder Colorado, 1991

- McTaggert, Lynn, *What Doctors Don't Tell You,* Thorson's, London, 1996 pgs 244-245,   pages 155-156

- Meinig, George, *Root Canal Cover-Up*, Bion
  Publishing, Ojai, California, 1996

- Micklem R.D., Carcinosin, A compendium of
  References, 1988

- Miller, R. Gibson. *Relationship of Remedies with
  Duration of Action*, B. Jain Publishers, reprint 1997

- Morrison, Roger, M.D., *Desktop Guide to keynotes
  and confirmatory symptoms*, Hahnemann Clinic
  Publishing, Albany, California, 1993

- Murphy, Robin, Homeopathic Medical Repertory, A
  Modern Alphabetical Repertory, Hahnemann
  Academy of North America, 1993

- Murray, Michael, Pizzorno Joseph, *The Encyclopedia
  of Natural Medicine*. Prima Publishing, Rocklin,
  California, 1991

- Ramsay, Melvin, *Myalgic Encephalomyelitis and
  Postviral Fatigue States*, Gower Medical Publishing,
  London, 1988

- Rosenbaum and Susser, *Solving the Puzzle of Chronic
  Fatigue Syndrome*, Life Sciences Press, Tacoma WA,
  1992

- Schimmel, Helmut. *Functional Medicine*. Karl F. Haug Verlag, Heidelberg, Germany, 1996

- Tyler ML *Homeopathic Drug Pictures*, B. Jain Publishers Ltd., New Delhi, 1980

- Vithoulkas, George. *The Science of Homeopathy*, Thorsons Publishers, Northampton, England, 1980

- Walter, Hughes, Gairdner, et al, "Three Years of Progress," *Persistent Virus Disease   Research Foundation*, Beaconsfield, Bucks, 1996

- Watson, Ian. *A Guide to the Methodologies of Homeopathy*. Cutting Edge Publications, Kendall, Cumbria, England, 1991

- Whitmont, Edward, *Psyche and Substance*, North Atlantic Books, Berkeley, California, 1980

- Van Straten, Michael. *The Natural Health Consultant*, Ebury Press, London, 1987

- Vithoukas, G. *A New Model of Health and Disease* North Atlantic Books, 1992

- Voge and Markell, *Medical Parasitology*, 6th Edition, W.B. Saunders Co., Philadelphia, 1986

RECOMMENDED READING

Introductory:

1) *The Family Guide To Homeopathy*, Alain Horvilleur, M.D., Health And Homeopathy Publishing, Inc.; Virginia, U.S.A.; 1986

2) *Everybody's Guide to Homeopathic Medicines,* Stephen Cummings and Dana Ullman, Jeremy P. Tarcher, Los Angeles, Ca. U.S.A.; 2004

3) *Homeopathic Medicine, A Doctor's Guide to Remedies For Common Ailments*, Trevor Smith, M.D., Healing Arts Press, Rochester, VT. 1989

4) *Impossible Cure: The Promise of Homeopathy Paperback,* Amy Lansky, R.L. Ranch Press, 2003

5) *The Complete Guide to Homeopathy: The Principles and Practice of Treatment*, Andrew Lockie, DK Adult, New York, 1995

6) *Encyclopedia of Homeopathy*, Andrew Lockie, DK, New York, 2006

Theory:

1) *The Science Of Homeopathy*, George Vithoulkas, Grove Press, Inc, New York; 1980

Professional:

1) *Lectures On Materia Medica*, James Tyler Kent, B. Jain Publishers, New Delhi, India; 1993 Reprint Edition

2) *Homeopathic Drug Pictures*, M.L. Tyler, B. Jain Publishers, New Delhi, India; 1980

3) *Allen's Key-notes Rearranged & Classified: With Leading Remedies of the Materia Medica & Bowel Nosodes,* Henry Clay Allen, B Jain Pub Pvt Ltd; New Delhi, India, June 2006

4) *Bowel Nosodes,* John Paterson, B. Jain Publishers, New Delhi, India; January, 1998

Sources for Homeopathic Books

Homeopathic Educational Services
2124 Kittredge St., Berkeley, CA 94704
800-359-9051
510-649-0294
mail@homeopathic.com
http://www.homeopathic.com/index.html

Minimum Price Homeopathic Books
250 H Street, PO Box 2187, Blaine, WA 98231
800-663-8272
Fax: 604-597-8304
orders@minimum.com
http://www.minimum.com/

<u>Minerva Homoeopathic Books</u>
Bratton Road, West Ashton, Trowbridge, Wiltshire
BA14 6AZ
Telephone +44 1225 760003
minervabks@aol.com
http://www.minervabooks.com/

ABOUT THE AUTHOR

Diane Solomon B.S., DHM, Dip.I.O.N., is a nutritionist and homeopath trained in London at the prestigious Institute of Optimum Nutrition and The British Institute of Homeopathy. Although empowered by her training in nutrition, adding the modality of homeopathy/energy healing to her practice resulted in even greater success and health for her clients. She states that homeopathy is "the most powerful healing mechanism we have."

Although she retired from practice in order to focus on writing, Diane helped thousands of people. She employed a combination of nutrients, herbs, homeopathic remedies, and diet and lifestyle recommendations, designing a personal plan for each person. She routinely worked with women's issues such as perimenopause and menopausal problems, Chronic Fatigue Syndrome, asthma and allergies, migraines, and arthritis. In her extensive practice she also enjoyed great success with many other problems such as eczema and psoriasis, fibromyalgia, ADD and ADHD, OCD, and much more.

Diane lives in Hillsborough County, New Hampshire, with her husband Mark. She writes novels, books on health, and edits and occasionally ghost-writes for others who as she puts it, "have something great to say!"

For more information, go to www.EloquentRascals.com

If you enjoy this book, and find it useful, please consider posting a review on Amazon. Then I can reach even more people who may need this information. Thanks!

AMAZON REVIEW:
http://www.amazon.com/CHRONIC-FATIGUE-SYNDROME-homeopathic-treatment-ebook/dp/B0186JMJSC/

(This page left blank for your notes)

ENDNOTE REFERENCES

1 Jason, LA, and JA, Richman, et.al. "A Community Based Study of Chronic Fatigue Syndrome." Archives of Internal Medicine 159.18 (2009): 2129-137. US National Library of Medicine, National Institutes of Health. Web. March 10, 2015 <http://www.ncbi.nlm.nih.gov/pubmed/10527290>.

2 "Beyond Myalgic Encephalomyelitis/Chronic Fatigue Syndrome: Redefining an Illness." Institute of Medicine. 10 Feb. 2015. Web. 15 Mar. 2015. <http://iom.nationalacademies.org/Reports/2015/ME-CFS.aspx>.

3 US National Library of Medicine Press Release, Feb 10, 2015. Web May 25, 2015.
http://www.nlm.nih.gov/medlineplus/news/fullstory_150867.html

4 CFIDS Association, "Yuppie Flu Is Dead." Townsend Letter for Doctors Aug/Sept 1995 (1995): 145/146. Print.

5 Ali, Majid, MD. The Canary and Chronic Fatigue: Reversing Chronic Fatigue" Life Span Press, Denville, New Jersey, 1995

6 Rosati, Peggy Allen, "Chronic Fatigue Syndrome: Implications for Women and Their Health Care Providers During the Childbearing Years." J Midwifery Womens Health 53(4) (2008):289-301. Web. June 1 2015. < http://www.medscape.com/viewarticle/576986_2 >.

7 R.T. Clement, M.D., "Chronic Fatigue Syndrome," syllabus BHII/HEEL conference, New York, April 1997, page 3

8 Ibid.

9 US Center for Disease Control and Prevention. "CFS toolkit for health care professionals" Atlanta, GA: Department of Health and Human Services. Web. December 11, 2007.
http:// www.cdc.gov/cfs/toolkit.htm

10 "Chronic Fatigue Syndrome: Who's at Risk?" Centers for Disease Control and Prevention. Web Oct 2 2015.
http://www.cdc.gov/cfs/causes/risk-groups.html

11 Ibid.

12 Ibid.

13 Zimmer, J. "Treating CFIDS: The Clinician's View," CFIDS
Chronicle, Summer 1995

14 Bombadier, CH, and D, Et Al Buchwald. "Outcome and Prognosis
of Patients with Chronic Fatigue vs Chronic Fatigue Syndrome."
Archives of Internal Medicine 155 (19) (1995): 2105-10. Print.

15 Tucker, Miriam, "Wrong Name, Real Illness." January 8, 2015.
Medscape Rheumatology. Web
http://www.medscape.com/viewarticle/837577

16 Ibid.

17 Salit IE. "Precipitating factors for the chronic fatigue syndrome." J
Psychiatric Res 31:1, (1997)59-65

18 "Chronic Fatigue Syndrome: A Definition." Mayo Clinic. Web. 10
Sept. 2015. <http://www.mayoclinic.org/diseases-conditions/chronic-
fatigue-syndrome/basics/definition/CON-20022009?p=1 Web. April
17 2015:>.

19 Chaitow, Leon. Masterclass, "Chronic Fatigue Syndrome and
Fibromyalgia." International Journal of Alternative and
Complementary Medicine, June 1995, page 12

20 Tucker, Miriam, "Wrong Name, Real Illness." January 8, 2015.
Medscape Rheumatology. Web
http://www.medscape.com/viewarticle/837577

21 Ibid.

22 CDC "Epidemiological studies of chronic fatigue syndrome at the
CDC." Centers for Disease Control, Atlanta, Georgia, statement
regarding Chronic Fatigue Syndrome: 1996 http://www.cdc.gov/cfs/

23 Bou-Holaigah, Rowe P.C. et al, "Is Neurally-Mediated
Hypotension an Unrecognized Cause of Chronic Fatigue?" The Lancet
345: 8950;623 (2) (1995) Print.

24 CDC Centers for Disease Control and Prevention. "Chronic Fatigue
Syndrome." Web. May 21 2015
http://www.cdc.gov/cfs/causes/index.html

25 Collin, Jonathan, MD. "Chronic Fatigue, Mycotoxins, Abnormal
Clotting and Other notes," Townsend Letter For Doctors, #157/8
Aug/Sept 1996 page 4

26 Marchesani, R, "Observations of Dr. Burke Cunha," Infectious
Disease News, Vol 5 No 11 November 1992. Print.

27 Chaitow, L, "Reports and Comments on the latest worldwide medical research," International Journal of Complementary Medicine, May (1994): 32. Print

28 Smit, Alta, "Chronic Fatigue syndrome- A Homotoxicological View," Biologische Medizin; 1996 August; 159-65

29 Levine PH, Atherton M, et al. "An approach to studies of cancer subsequent to clusters of chronic fatigue syndrome: use of data from the Nevada State Cancer Registry." Clinical Infectious Diseases. 18 (supp) 1: S49-53, (1994) Jan

30 Peterson PK Sirr SA, et al. "Effects of mild exercise on cytokines and cerebral blood flow in chronic fatigue syndrome patients." Clinical and Diagnostic Laboratory Immunology. 1 (2) : 222-6, 1994 Mar

31 Rosenbaum, Susser. Solving the Puzzle of Chronic Fatigue, Life Sciences Press, Tacoma WA, 1992

32 Caligiuri M, Murray c, et al. "Phenotypic and functional deficiency of natural killer cells in patients with chronic fatigue syndrome." Journal of Immunology (1987 Nov) 139 (10): 3306-13

33 Baker E, et al. "Immunologic abnormalities associated with chronic fatigue syndrome." Clinical Infectious Diseases 1994; 18 (supp 1) 136-41

34 Levy JA. "Viral studies of chronic fatigue syndrome-introduction." Clinical Infectious Diseases 1994; 18 (supp 1): 117-20

35 Swanink CM, Vercoulen JH, et al. "All lymphocyte subsets, apoptosis, and cytokines in patients with chronic fatigue syndrome." J Infectious Diseases (1996 Feb) 173 (2); 460-3

36 Bates DW, Buchwald D, et al. Clinical laboratory test findings I patients with chronic fatigue syndrome. Arch. Int. Med. (1995 Jan 9) 155 (1): 97-103

37 Lloyd A.R., Wakefield, D et al. "Immunological abnormalities in the chronic fatigue syndrome." Med. J. Aust. (1989 August 7) 151 (3): 122-4

38 Courage, K, "Baffling Chronic Fatigue Syndrome Set for Diagnostic Overhaul, Scientific American, May 16, 2014. http://www.scientificamerican.com/article/baffling-chronic-fatigue-syndrome-set-for-diagnostic-overhaul/ Web July 3 2014.

39 Saiki, Kawai T, et al, Identification of marker genes for differential diagnosis of chronic fatigue syndrome. Mol Med. 2008 Sep-Oct;14(9-10):599-607. doi: 10.2119/2007-00059

40 Mawle,C, Nisenbaum,R., et al. "Seroepidemiology of Chronic Fatigue Syndrome: A Case-Control Study." Clinical Infectious Diseases, vol 21, 1997, pages 1286-1389

41 Reyes, M, Dobbins, J. et al. "Risk Factors for Chronic Fatigue Syndrome: A Case-Control Study." Journal of Chronic Fatigue Syndrome, vol 2 (1996): 17-33

42 CDC Centers for Disease Control and Prevention. "Chronic Fatigue Syndrome." Web. May 21 2015
http://www.cdc.gov/cfs/causes/index.html

43 Ibid.

44 Lerner, A. Martin et al (2010). "An update on the management of glandular fever (infectious mononucleosis) and its sequelae caused by Epstein–Barr virus (HHV-4): new and emerging treatment strategies." Virus adaptation and treatment 2: 135 – 145. Web. Jun 2, 2015

45 Ibid.

46 A.H Rowe, Food Allergy- Its manifestation and control. Marcel
Dekker, Inc. New York. 2005: 39

47 Schimmel, Helmut. Functional Medicine. Karl F. Haug Verlag,
Heidelberg, Germany, 1996, page 27

48 Steckelbrook, V., Hubner, F. "Homeopathic Treatment in
Obstetrics." Biomedical Therapy, June 1998, page 218

49 Enbergs, H. DVM. "The Effect of Selected Potentiated Suis Organ
Preparations and Traumeel on Phagocyte and Lymphocyte Activity."
Biomedical Therapy, April 1998, Pages 178-184

50 Schimmel, Helmut. Functional Medicine. Karl F. Haug Verlag,
Heidelberg, Germany, 1996, page 15

51 Voll, Reinhold, Fundamentals of Electroacupuncture, Medizinisch
Literarische Verlagsgesellschaft , Uelzen,   Germany, 1980, page 20

52 John Paterson, Bowel Nosodes, B. Jain Publishers, New Delhi,
India; January, 1998

53 Makewell, de Ai-ling, "Bowel nosodes: A group of neglected remedies." August 2006. Web http://www.interhomeopathy.org/fr-bowel-nosodes-a-group-of-neglected-remedies

54 Henry Clay Allen, Allen's Key-notes Rearranged & Classified: With Leading Remedies of the Materia Medica & Bowel Nosodes, June 2006 B Jain Pub Pvt Ltd; 10 Lrg edition

55 Voll, Reinhold, Fundamentals of Electroacupuncture, Medizinisch Literarische Verlagsgesellschaft, Uelzen, Germany, 1980 pages 56-72

56 Schimmel, Helmut. Functional Medicine. Karl F. Haug Verlag, Heidelberg, Germany, 1996, page 106

57 Ibid. pages 91-117

58 Meinig, George, Root Canal Cover-Up, Bion Publishing, Ojai, California, 2008, page 140

59 Huggins, Hal, DDS. It's All in Your Head. The Link between Mercury Amalgams and Illness. Avery Publishing Group, Garden City Park, New York, 1993, pages 28-29

60 McTaggert, Lynne. What Doctors Don't Tell You, Thorsons
Publishers, London 2005 pages 240-255

61 Ibid. page 238

62 Ibid. page 249

63 "Giardiasis Surveillance — United States." CDC Centerr for
Disease Control and Prevention, Morbidity and Mortality, Weekly
Report, May 1, 2015 2011–2012 Web May 20 2015
http://www.cdc.gov/mmwr/preview/mmwrhtml/ss6403a2.htm

64 Yutsis, P., and Walker, M. The Downhill Syndrome, If Nothing's
Wrong, Why do I Feel so Bad? Avery Publishing Group, Inc 1997

65 Ibid.

66 Casura L, "Sick of Being Patient. Part Two. Why Alternative
Medicine offers more hope than conventional in treating CFS."
Townsend Letter for Doctors 156 July 1996, pages 54-55, 64

67 Walker Morton, "Protozoa and Worms that Live Inside US".
Explore, For the Professional, Vol 8, No 2, 1997, page 20

68 Ibid. p 21

69 Buttram, Harold, MD, "The National Childhood Vaccine Injury
Act- A Critique." Townsend Letter for Doctors, #184; October 1998,
p66-69

70 Murphy, Robin, N.D., Homeopathic Medical Repertory,
Hahnemann Academy of North America, Pagosa Springs, Colorado,
1993 page 559

71 "The evidence for homeopathy: There is a growing body of clinical
evidence to show that homeopathy has a positive effect." British
Homeoapthic Association. Web August 12 2015
http://www.britishhomeopathic.org/evidence/the-evidence-for-
homeopathy/ Web. July 6 2015

72 Peter Tyson Dogs' Dazzling Sense of Smell, Nova ScienceNow.
Oct 10, 2012. http://www.pbs.org/wgbh/nova/nature/dogs-sense-of-
smell.html. Accessed Nov 19 2015

73 Chikramane PS, Suresh AK et al. "Extreme homeopathic dilutions
retain starting materials: A nanoparticulate perspective."

Homeopathy. 2010 Oct;99(4):231-42. doi:
10.1016/j.homp.2010.05.006. Accessed Nov 20 2015

74 Bell IR, Koithan M "A model for homeopathic remedy effects: low
dose nanoparticles, allostatic cross-adaptation, and time-dependent
sensitization in a complex adaptive system." BMC Comp Altern Med,
2012 Oct 22;12:191. doi: 10.1186/1472-6882-12-191.

75 Chikramane PS1, Kalita D et al. "Why extreme dilutions reach non-
zero asymptotes: a nanoparticulate hypothesis based on froth
flotation." Langmuir. 2012 Nov 13;28(45):15864-75. doi:
10.1021/la303477s. Epub 2012 Nov 1. Accessed Nov 20 2015

76 "The evidence base," Faculty of Homeopathy. Web. July 6 2015
http://www.facultyofhomeopathy.org/research/

77 El Dib RP, Atallah AN, et al. "Mapping the Cochrane evidence for
decision making in health care." Journal of Evaluation in Clinical
Practice; (2007) 13:689–692.

78 Eskinazi D, Muehsam D. "Is the scientific publishing of
complementary and alternative medicine objective?" J Altern
Complement Med. 1999 Dec;5(6):587-94. Accessed Nov 15, 2015

79 Dana Ullman, "The Swiss Government's Remarkable Report on
Homeopathic Medicine" Huffington Post, 02/15/2012 Accessed Nov
15 2015

80 Awdry, Robert. "Homeopathy and chronic fatigue- the search for
proof." Journal of Alternative and Complementary Medicine, Feb
1996 page 19

81 Ibid. page 21

82 Ibid., page 21

83 Weatherley Jones ,E,.Thompson, E.A. "Placebo Control Trial in
CAM . The placebo controlled trial as a test of complementary and
alternative medicine; observations from research experience of
individualized homeopathy treatment." Homeopath .vol.93, (4) (2004)
-p.186-189

84 Awdry, Robert Homeopathy and chronic fatigue- the search for
proof. Journal of Alternative and Complementary Medicine, March
1996 page 13

85 Rude RK, Ross AC, et al. Magnesium. In Modern Nutrition in Health and Disease. 11th ed. Baltimore, Mass: Lippincott Williams & Wilkins; 2012:159-75.

86 King D, Mainous A, et al. "Dietary magnesium and C-reactive protein levels." J Am Coll Nutr. 2005 Jun 24(3):166-71.

87 National Health and Nutrition Examination Survey (NHANES) of 2005–2006, National Institues of Health: http://ods.od.nih.gov/factsheets/Magnesium-HealthProfessional/ Web. June 1 2015

88 Chaitow, Leon. Post Viral Fatigue Syndrome, Everyman, Dents, 1990

89 Hoffman, Ronald, Tired all the Time, Simon and Simon, N.Y., N.Y., 1993 page 219

90 Arnaud, Maurice, "Update on the assessment of magnesium status" British Journal of Nutrition (2008), 99, Suppl. 3, S24–S36 Web. Accessed Nov 10 2015

91 Kirk Hamilton, Clinical Pearls in Nutrition and Preventive
Medicine, ITServices, Health Associates Medical Group, Sacramento,
California, 1993 page111

92 Levy JA. "Viral studies of chronic fatigue syndrome-introduction."
Clinical Infectious Diseases 18 (supp 1) (1994): 117-20

93 Kelley KW, Bluth'e RM, Dantzer R, Zhou JH, Shen WH, Johnson
RW, Broussard SR. Cytokine-induced sickness behavior. Brain Behav
Immun 2003;17:S112–S118. 33. de Lange FP, .CR, Dwyer JM.
Immunological References 151.

94 Clement, RT. "Chronic Fatigue Syndrome." Heel/BHI convention
on CFS, New York, March 1997

95 Gow JW. Et al. "Studies on enteroviruses in patients with CFS"
Clinical Infectious Diseases 18 (supp 1) (1994): 126-33

96 Dharam V, Ablashi et al. "Viruses and Chronic Fatigue Syndrome:
Current Status." Journal of Chronic Fatigue Syndrome 1 (2) (1995): 3-
22

97 Heneine W et al. "Lack of Evidence for infection with known retroviruses in patients with CFS." Clinical Infectious Diseases 18 (supp 1) (1994): 121-5

98 Smith RA "Contamination of clinical specimens with MLV-encoding nucleic acids: implications for XMRV and other Candidate human retroviruses" (PDF). Retrovirology 7(1): 112. Dec 2010 doi:10.1186/1742-4690-7-112. PMC 3022688.PMID 21171980

99 Menéndez-Arias L, "Evidence and controversies on the role of XMRV in prostate cancer and chronic fatigue syndrome". Rev. Med. Virol. 21 (1): 3–17. Jan 2011. doi:10.1002/rmv.673.PMID 21294212.

100 Suhaldonik RJ et al. "Upregulation of the 2-5-A synthetase RNAse antiviral pathway associated with CFS." Clinical Infectious Diseases 18 (supp 1) (1994):96-104

101 Pantry, S, Medveczky, M. "Persistent human herpesvirus-6 infection in patients with an inherited form of the virus; " Journal of Medical Virology; July 2013, DOI: 10.1002/jmv.23685 Web July 12 2015

102 Pall ML, "Common etiology of posttraumatic stress disorder, fibromyalgia, chronic fatigue syndrome and multiple chemical sensitivity via elevated nitric oxide/peroxynitrite," Med Hypotheses Aug;57(2) (2001):139-45

103 Pall ML, Satterle JD., "Elevated nitric oxide/peroxynitrite mechanism for the common etiology of multiple chemical sensitivity, chronic fatigue syndrome, and posttraumatic stress disorder." Ann N Y Acad Sci Mar;933 (2001):323-9

104 "Chronic Fatigue Syndrome: Causes." Center for Disease Control and Prevention. 14 May 2012. Web. 5 June 2015. <http://www.cdc.gov/cfs/causes/>.

105 Hilgers, A., Frank,J., "Chronic Fatigue Syndrome: immune dysfunction, role of pathogens and toxic agents and neurological and cardial changes," Weiner Medizinische Wochenschrift 144 (16) (1994): 399-406. Print.

106 VanElzakker, MB. "Chronic Fatigue Syndrome from Vagus Nerve Infection: A Psychoneuroimmunological Hypothesis." Med Hypotheses Sep;81(3) (2013): 414-23. Pub Med. US National Library

of Medicine, National Institutes of Health. Web. 4 Oct. 2015.
<http://www.ncbi.nlm.nih.gov/pubmed/23790471>.

107 Lloyd A, et al. "Cytokine production and fatigue in patients with
CFS and healthy control subjects in response to exercise." Clinical
Infectious Diseases 18 (supp 1) (1994): 142-46

108 Patarca R et al. "Dysregulated expression of tumor necrosis factor
in CFS: interrelations with cellular sources and patterns of soluble
mediator expression." Clinical Infectious Diseases 18 (supp 1) (1994):
147-53

109 Johnson, C. "One Theory To Explain Them All? The Vagus
Nerve Infection Hypothesis for Chronic Fatigue Syndrome."
Simmaron Research. 13 Dec. 2013. Web. 14 Sept. 2015.
<http://simmaronresearch.com/2013/12/one-theory-explain-vagus-
nerve-infection-chronic-fatigue-syndrome/#sthash.zrTliogQ.dpuf>.

110 von Mikecz A, Konstaninov K, et al. "High frequency of
autoantibodies to insoluble cellular antigens in patients with chronic
fatigue syndrome." Arthritis and Rheumatism. 40(2): 295-305, 1997
Feb

111 Konstaninov K. von Mikecz A et al. "Autoantibodies to nuclear envelope antigens in chronic fatigue syndrome." Journal of Clinical Investigation. 98 (8): 1888-96, 1996, Oct 15

112 Yoshida, S, Gerswin ME. "Autoimmunity and selected environmental factors of disease induction." Semin. Arthritis. Rheum. 1993; 22 (6): 399-419

113 Reichlin SI. "Neuroendocrine-immune interactions." New England Journal of Medicine. 1993; 21: 1246-52

114 Hilgers, A., Frank, J., "Chronic Fatigue Syndrome: immune dysfunction, role of pathogens and toxic agents and neurological and cardial changes," Weiner Medizinische Wochenschrift 144 (16): 399-406, 1994

115 Nicholson, Garth, et al. "Diagnosis and Treatment of Chronic Mycoplasmal Infections in Fibromyalgia and Chronic Fatigue Syndrome: Relationship to Gulf War Illness." Biomedical Therapy, Vol. XVI No. 4, October 1998, page 266

116 Nicholson, Garth, et al. "Chronic Fatigue illness and Operation Desert Storm." J Occup Environ. Med (38) (1996):14-16

117 Nijs J1, Nicolson GL, et. al. "High prevalence of Mycoplasma infections among European chronic fatigue syndrome patients. Examination of four Mycoplasma species in blood of chronic fatigue syndrome patients." FEMS Immunol Med Microbiol. 2002 Nov 15;34(3):209-14.

118 Baseman, JB, Tully, JG. "Mycoplasmas: Sophisticated, re-emerging, and burdened by their notoriety." Emerging Infectious Disease. 1997 (3): 21-32

119 Nicholson, Garth, et al. "Diagnosis and Treatment of Chronic Mycoplasmal Infections in Fibromyalgia and Chronic Fatigue Syndrome: Relationship to Gulf War Illness." Biomedical Therapy, Vol. XVI No. 4, October 1998, page 266

120 Nicholson, Garth. Chronic infections as a common etiology for many patients with Chronic Fatigue Syndrome, Fibromyalgia Syndrome, and Gulf War Illness. Intern. Journal Med. 1998 (1): 42-46

121 Nicholson, G, Nicolson, NL et al. "Mycoplasmal infections and Chronic Fatigue Illness (Gulf War Illness) associated with deployment to Operation Desert Storm." Intern. Journal Med. 1998 (1):80-92

122 Ibid.

123 Bou-Holaigah I, Rowe PC, et al. "The relationship between
neurally mediated hypotension and the chronic fatigue syndrome."
JAMA 274 (12) : 961-7, 1995 Sep 27

124 van Houdenhove B, et al. "Does high "action-proneness" make
people more vulnerable to chronic fatigue syndrome?" Journal of
Psychosomatic Research 39 (5) 633-40, 1995, Jul

125 Hoffman, R, MD. Tired all the Time. Simon and Schuster, New
York1993: 213

126 Ibid.

127 Panerai AE, Vecchiet J. et al. "Peripheral blood mononuclear cell
beta-endorphin concentration is decreased in chronic fatigue syndrome
and fibromyalgia but not in depression: preliminary report." Clin J
Pain 2002 Jul-Aug;18(4):270-3

128 Casura L, "Sick of Being Patient. Why Alternative Medicine
offers more hope than conventional in treating CFS." Townsend Letter
for Doctors 155 June 1996: 37

129 Buchwald D et al. "A Chronic Illness characterized by fatigue, neurologic and immune disorders and active HHV 6 infection." Annals of Internal Medicine 1992; 116; 103-13

130 Ibid.

131 Sc Cook DB, Lange G, et al. "Relationship of brain MRI abnormalities and physical functional status in chronic fatigue syndrome." Int J Neuroscience 2001 Mar;107(1-2):1-6hwartz

132 RB Garada BM et al. "Detection of intracranial abnormalities in patients with chronic fatigue syndrome: Comparison of MR imaging and SPECT." American Journal of Roentgenology. 164 (4); 935-41, 1994 Apr.

133 Costa DC et al. "Brain stem and SPECT studies in normals, ME/CFS and depression." Nucl. Med. Commun 1992; 302: 1567

134 Van Houdenhove B, Neerinckx E, et al. "Daily hassles reported by chronic fatigue syndrome and fibromyalgia patients in tertiary care: a controlled quantitative and qualitative study." Psychother Psychosom 2002 Jul-Aug;71(4):207-13

135 Nater, UM1, Maloney E, et al. "Attenuated morning salivary cortisol concentrations in a population-based study of persons with chronic fatigue syndrome and well controls." J Clin Endocrinol Metab. 2008 Mar;93(3):703-9. Epub 2007 Dec 26.

136 Nater UM1, Youngblood LS, et al. " Alterations in diurnal salivary cortisol rhythm in a population-based sample of cases with chronic fatigue syndrome." Psychosom Med. 2008 Apr;70(3):298-305. doi: 10.1097/PSY.0b013e3181651025. Epub 2008 Mar 31.

137 Cleare AJ, Blair D, et al. "Urinary free cortisol in chronic fatigue syndrome." Am J Psychiatry 2001 Apr;158(4):641-3

138 Ehlert U, Gaab J, et al. "Psychoneuroendocrinological contributions to the etiology of depression, posttraumatic stress disorder, and stress-related bodily disorders: the role of the hypothalamus-pituitary-adrenal axis." Biol Psychol 2001 Jul-Aug;57(1-3):141-52

139 Cleare AJ, O'Keane V, et al. "Plasma leptin in chronic fatigue syndrome and a placebo-controlled study of the effects of low-dose hydrocortisone on leptin secretion." Clin Endocrinol (Oxf) 2001 Jul;55(1):113-9

140 Cleare AJ, Miell J, et al. "Hypothalamo-pituitary-adrenal axis
dysfunction in chronic fatigue syndrome, and the effects of low-dose
hydrocortisone therapy." J Clin Endocrinol Metab 2001
Aug;86(8):3545-54

141 Bell, DS. "Chronic fatigue syndrome update. Findings now point
to a CNS involvement." Harvard Medical School . Postgraduate
Medicine. 1996 (6): 73-6, 79-81, 1994, Nov 1

142 Demitrack MA, Dale JK, et al. "Evidence for impaired activation
of the hypothalamic-pituitary-adrenal axis I patients with chronic
fatigue syndrome." Journal of Clinical Endocrine Metab. (1991 Dec)
73 (6): 1224-34

143 Cleare, Anthony, Wessely, Simon, "Chronic Fatigue Syndrome:
A Stress Disorder?" British Journal of Hospital Medicine, 1996: 55
(9) : 571-574

144 Visser JT, De Kloet ER, et al. "Altered glucocorticoid regulation
of the immune response in the chronic fatigue syndrome." Ann N Y
Acad Sci 2000;917:868-75

145 Rosenbaum and Susser, Solving the Puzzle of Chronic Fatigue
Syndrome. Life Sciences Press, Tacoma WA, 1992

146 Regland B, Andersson M, et al. "Increased concentrations of
homocysteine in the cerebrospinal fluid in patients with fibromyalgia
and chronic fatigue syndrome." Scand J Rhematol, 1997, 26:4, 301-7

147 Kuratsane H et al. "Acetylcarnitine deficiency in chronic fatigue
syndrome." Clinical Infectious Diseases 1994; 18 (supp 1): 62-7

148 Barnes PRJ et al. "Skeletal muscle bioenergetics in chronic fatigue
syndrome." Neurosurgery and Psychiatry 1993; 56: 679-83

149 Plioplys AV. Plioplys S. "Serum levels of carnitine in chronic
fatigue syndrome: clinical correlation." Neuropsychobiology. 32(3):
132-8, 1995

150 Plioplys AV. Plioplys S. "Amantadine and L-carnitine treatment
in Chronic Fatigue Syndrome." Neuropsychobiology, 1997, 35:1, 16-
23

151 Chaitow, Leon. Post Viral Fatigue Syndrome, Everyman, Dents,
1989

152 Hoffman, R, MD. Tired all the Time. Simon and Schuster, New York1993: 219

153 Walker, Morton. "Metallic Toxicity as a Cause of the Downhill Syndrome." Townsend Letter for Doctors. (160) November 1996 pages 116-122

154 Ibid., page 130

155 Bennett AL, Mayes DM et al. "Somatomedin C levels I patients with chronic fatigue syndrome." J Psychiatric Res, 1997 Jan, 31:1, 91-6

156 Buchwald, D, Garrity, D, "Comparison of patients with CFS, FMS, and MCS." Archives of Internal Medicine 154 (18):2049-2053: 1994

157 Ibid.

158 Gomborone JE, Gorard DA, et al. "Prevalence of irritable bowel syndrome in chronic fatigue." J R Coll Physicians. London, 1996 Nov, 30:6, 512-3

159 A.H Rowe, "Allergic toxemia and migraine due to food allergy."
California and West Medical Journal 33:785, Nov 1930

160 A.H Rowe, Food Allergy- Its manifestation and control. Marcel
Dekker, Inc. New York. 2005: 47, 250

161 A Venket Rao, Alison C Bested, etc al. "A randomized, double-
blind, placebo-controlled pilot study of a probiotic in emotional
symptoms of chronic fatigue syndrome," Gut Pathog. 2009; 1: 6. Web
Aug 28 2015
<http://www.ncbi.nlm.nih.gov/pmc/articles/PMC2664325/

162 Bailey MT et al. "Prenatal stress alters bacterial colonization of
the gut in infant monkeys". J Pediatr Gastroenterol Nutr 2004,
38:414-421. Print

163 Bailey MT, Coe C. "Maternal separation disrupts the integrity of
the intestinal microflora in infant rhesus monkeys." Dev Psychobiol
1999, 35: 146-155. Print

164 Lakhan SE, Kirchgessner A." Gut inflammation in chronic fatigue
syndrome". Nutr Metab (Lond) 2010, 7: 79. Print.

165 Lerner AM, Beqaj SH, et al. "IgM serum antibodies to Epstein-Barr virus are uniquely present in a subset of patients with the chronic fatigue syndrome" In Vivo. 2004 Mar-Apr;18(2):101-6.

166 Hoffman, Ronald, Tired all the Time, Simon and Simon, N.Y., 1993 page 215

167   Gilje, A." What Is Happening with the Research into ME and Rituximab?" 12 Mar. 2012. Invest In ME.org Web. 5 Sept. 2015. <http://www.investinme.org/InfoCentre-Library-NMEA-Newsletter-1203.htm>.

168 "Further Evidence of Rituximab's Effectiveness in Treating ME/CFS | PlosOne Publish Results of Phase 2 Trial." ME Association. 1 July 2015. Web. 13 Oct. 2015.
<http://www.meassociation.org.uk/2015/07/comments-further-evidence-of-rituximabs-effectiveness-in-treating-mecfs-plosone-publish-results-of-phase-2-trial-1-july-2015/>.

169 Øystein Flug, et al. "Further evidence of Rituximab's effectiveness in treating ME/CFS | PlosOne publish results" PlosOne July 1 2015. Web. http://www.meassociation.org.uk/2015/07/comments-further-evidence-of-rituximabs-effectiveness-in-treating-mecfs-plosone-publish-results-of-phase-2-trial-1-july-2015/

170 "The Biggest Chronic Fatigue Syndrome Treatment Trial Begins: Fluge/Mella On Rituximab - Simmaron Research." Simmaron Research. 20 Jan. 2015. Web. 2 Oct. 2015. http://simmaronresearch.com/2015/01/chronic-fatigue-syndrome-rituximab-fluge-mella/

171 Ali, Majid, M.D., The Canary and Chronic Fatigue: Reversing Chronic Fatigue. 2nd Edition, Life Span Press, Denville, NJ 1995

172 Hoffman, Ronald, Tired all the Time, Simon and Simon, N.Y., N.Y., 1993 page 1990

173 Fulcher KY, White Pd. "Randomized controlled trial of graded exercise in patients with chronic fatigue syndrome." BMJ, 1997 June, 314: 7095, 1647-522

174 White PD, Goldsmith KA, Johnson AL, et al; "PACE trial
management group. Comparison of adaptive pacing therapy, cognitive
behaviour therapy, graded exercise therapy, and specialist medical
care for chronic fatigue syndrome (PACE): a randomised trial."
Lancet. 2011;377:823-
836. http://www.ncbi.nlm.nih.gov/pmc/articles/PMC3065633/ Access
ed June 13, 2015.

Made in the USA
Columbia, SC
22 September 2018